G000123523

Confident Birth

Confident Birth

■ First published in Swedish as *Föda utan rädsla* by Bokförlaget Bonnier Existens.
■ This revised English edition first published by Pinter & Martin Ltd 2012

■ © Susanna Heli 2009, 2012

■ Translated by Joanna Tisell ■ Design and illustrations Eva-Jo Hancock

■ All rights reserved

■ ISBN 978-1-78066-040-0 ■ also available as ebook

■ The right of Susanna Heli to be identified as the author of this work has been asserted by her in accordance with the Copyright, Designs and Patent Act of 1988

■ British Library Cataloguing-in-Publication Data
A catalogue record for this book is available from the British Library

■ This book is sold subject to the condition that it shall not, by way of trade and otherwise, be lent, resold, hired out, or otherwise circulated without the publisher's prior consent in any form or binding or cover other than that in which it is published and without a similar condition being imposed on the subsequent purchaser.

■ Printed in the UK by TJ International Ltd, Padstow, Cornwall

■ This book has been printed on paper that is sourced and harvested from sustainable forests and is FSC accredited

Pinter & Martin Ltd
6 Effra Parade
London SW2 1PS

www.pinterandmartin.com

Confident Birth

SUSANNA HELI

pinter & martin

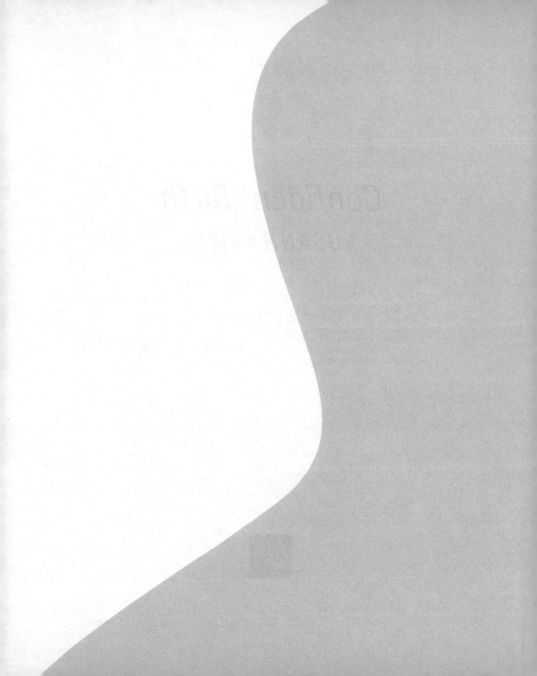

Contents

Introduction

I THOUGHT I WAS IN TOUCH WITH MY BODY. I thought I was well prepared to give birth. I could not have been more wrong. I would never have been able to imagine what giving birth was going to be like, the enormity of the force and how much it scared me. The pain was not at all what I had thought it was going to be like, and the power of it choked me. Suddenly, I did not want to give birth at all! I started to fight my own body. I tried talking to it, pleading with it to stop. I just wanted to escape, disappear and leave this reality. Without me being conscious of it, the fear took over completely. I was terrified when a new contraction started, and scared when the contraction ended since that meant a new one was on the way and I was concerned that I would not have the stamina to deal with it. Mostly I was simply scared for my life, without really knowing why. Fear had taken over my whole being and blocked everything else out.

In the midst of this struggle my partner tells me my midwife wants to talk to me over the phone. I yell at him, telling him I do not want to talk to anyone. In spite of this he puts the receiver to my ear. Her words flow out of the speaker, telling me I am only making it worse by hyperventilating and tensing the body, though I was not aware of doing any of this. She tells me I have two choices. I can either keep doing what I am doing and have a hard time, or I can listen to her. This is not a difficult choice to make. I start listening.

She helps me to breathe in a new way, softly and soundlessly, and tells me to let my body become heavier during the contractions and to let the birth happen. She says that I need to relax and let go, instead of tensing up.

Slowly I start taking her words in, and I stop fighting. Despite being scared, I let my body sink and my breath soften when the contraction starts. The contrast is startling and I decide there and then to start trusting my body. This is what my body is made for, and I know that I have everything it takes to be able to give birth to my baby.

This new attitude towards my own body turned out to make all the difference, and it opened up a new world. I realized that by letting go of fear, I could suddenly hear my body and help it to give birth. It did not make the process painless or easy; it did, however, help me to find my way back to my body. My body, in turn, did know how to give birth. I was able to use various movements, breathing exercises, relaxation techniques and sounds. I used the power of the mind to create positive images and words. These simple techniques gave me the strength to face the pain and fear of birth, and a few hours later I gave birth to my son.

After delivery I realized I would probably have kept hyperventilating if I had not been helped to change my breathing. I would never have known the difference it could make, and I would have assumed that the panic I felt was part of the process. This insight was so profound it made me want to help others to find their inner power.

I started working as a nurse's assistant on a labour ward. I quickly noticed a lot of women experiencing the same fear I had during labour. Over and over again I saw women showing signs of strong physical stress caused by fear when facing pain. Pain led to fear, fear led to stress and stress led to negative physical reactions, blocking the body by activating the flight-or-fight response. The women were hyperventilating, extremely tense and focusing only on the pain. Their shoulders were up high, their jaws were tight, and their voices were filled with panic. They could not rest or sleep. They were completely numbed by fear and it drained their focus and strength.

I started using the simple techniques I had used during my own birth to be able to break or shift the negative pattern the women were trapped in. Time and time again I witnessed woman upon woman being able to give birth without fear by using these techniques. I understood then it was not pain itself but fear that was the cause of the stress reactions blocking the body. Once the women learnt how to handle the fear they were able to face the birthing process from a different angle. The contractions were still painful, but the pain became less frightening. The women were able to find something within themselves – an inner power helping them to give birth.

The modern health care system seems to have forgotten the knowledge of how to use breathing and relaxation in childbirth, but I had stumbled upon their remarkable effects. These simple techniques were an important missing part of the puzzle for women to be able to get in touch with their inner ability to give birth. I realized it was the emotional part of birth I wanted to work with, not the medical. I started working as a doula. Doula means birth support. To get a deeper understanding of the emotional impact on the body I chose to go to university to get a degree in psychosomatic physiotherapy (physical therapy based on the connection between body and soul).

Many years and hundreds of births later I have discovered four effective and powerful tools to break stress and fear. You will get to know them in this book. They are: 'breathing', 'relaxation', 'sound', and 'the power of the mind'.

The book opens with a chapter on stress and fear, which aims to provide a deeper understanding of how we react to these sensations and suggests ways of dealing with them. To be able to work against fear it is necessary to understand the purpose of pain. That is why I have devoted a large part of the first chapter to the normal birth process.

The middle section of the book is the practical and specific part. Here I introduce the four tools – *breathing, relaxation, sound* and *the power of the mind*. I provide a thorough explanation of the tools using pictures, theory, birth stories and exercises. I then go on to explain how to use the tools during the different phases of birth. I also talk about the importance of rest and activity, and how they interplay.

To prevent fear, and to use the tools to their best advantage, a woman needs support during birth. Therefore, the third section of the book deals with the importance of support. Having support during childbirth is important whether or not you are in a relationship. This is why I have chosen to call the person who takes on this role the 'support person'. It could be a partner, a friend, a doula or a family member. This part of the book is directed both at the woman and her support person. It includes advice and suggestions on the best way to support a woman during labour. This section also looks at the healing power of touch and massage. The book ends with a short summary of all the techniques and instructions used to serve as a quick reference guide.

The book contains many different exercises which will help you to deepen your understanding of the various techniques and terms used. Practising the exercises during pregnancy is a good preparation for labour. Allowing yourself space to listen to and respond to your body is the foundation of this book. It is appropriate to start doing the exercises during the second half of your pregnancy. You can, however, choose to do them as you come across them while reading the book.

I wrote this book to help women handle the fear they might face during childbirth, so that it does not block the ability to give birth. I use the word fear to encapsulate negative emotions like doubt, horror, dejection, insecurity and aggression. These emotions can hinder the body from accessing its inner ability. They trigger negative chain reactions like the fight-or-flight response.

Dr. Grantly Dick-Read wrote the book *Childbirth Without Fear* back in 1942. I did not read the book until I had finished writing my book and was stunned by how much of the knowledge I had been writing about existed seventy years ago. I was simultaneously baffled at how little has changed since then. Years have gone by where we could have prevented a lot of suffering and many negative birth experiences. Therefore I see this book as an important continuation of the work of Dr. Dick-Read and others who have followed in his footsteps. Dr. Dick-Read thought that pain in itself was a result of fear. I believe pain is a natural part of childbirth. I do, on the other hand, think that fear enforces the experience of pain, making it more acute, negative and destructive. Fear is a warning signal to the body and it slows down and obstructs the birth process.

I do not think it is possible to give birth entirely without fear, but, by using the tools in this book, you will be able to lessen the fear and take control over it. When fear no longer takes all the focus and energy, you will be able to feel more secure, more involved in the process, and less scared. When the body ceases to see a threat, the pain will ease and become less destructive. When fear no longer blocks the body, the uterus can do its work and move the birth along.

The four tools and the techniques presented in this book can be used regardless of where the birth takes place. The tools are not affected by the surrounding circumstances, and it makes no difference whether or not any pain relief is used. My wish is that the tools will help women to feel involved, strong and participatory during birth and that they will give women the self-confidence to give birth.

I do not think there are any methods or tools that will work for all women. Every woman is unique. This is what makes childbirth so special. Find what works for you and use the book to inspire you to listen to your body, and go deeper than you thought possible. Leave all preconceptions behind about giving birth and whether or not you want to use pain medication. Be open-minded. Be brave and respect yourself. Seek the wisdom you already have deep inside your body. It will show you how to face pain and how to give birth to a baby. This inner voice only has one mission – to help you give birth.

Susanna Heli

SUSANNA HELI

1

Confident birth

The human body is an amazing instrument. Deep inside, a woman carries all the wisdom she will ever need to be able to give birth to a child. However, fear often gets in the way of you and your body, and stops you from accessing this ancient knowledge. This is due to the fact that fear itself activates stress hormones. These hormones exist to keep you safe. This is an ancient mechanism, and has been crucial to the survival of our species. But since we no longer encounter the same threatening situations we used to, this mechanism can get in the way of the birthing process. It may be challenging to change this response, since this is an internal struggle, which mostly takes place without you even realizing it. Fortunately, it is possible to manipulate this response and prevent fear from descending into a negative spiral. In this chapter you will learn to understand fear, its origin, how it affects you, and how to break the cycle of fear. When fear no longer stands in the way, consuming all the focus and energy, you will be free to access your inner power. This will help you to give birth.

Understanding fear

During labour, you will truly merge with your body. This is a connection that involves your most basic instincts, which you might have never encountered previously in your life. You leave the sphere you normally operate in and enter a new dimension, where your body takes over and knows just what to do. This is an organic process, and is part of the heritage your body carries. It is what you are made to do. But this does not automatically make childbirth easy or simple. The enormous physical workout that goes on inside of you is unlike anything you have ever faced before, and it can feel unnatural compared to what you experience in your everyday life. Therefore it is not strange or surprising if you get scared or overwhelmed.

To be able to overcome fear it is important to understand the purpose of pain, and to know how a natural and healthy birth proceeds, and what takes place in your body during the birthing process. You will learn more about your amazing body in this chapter. To be able to differentiate between reactions caused by a natural birthing process, as opposed to reactions caused by fear, you will need to know how the body reacts to fear. Sometimes, the confusion brought on by these sensations creates even more fear. You might think the physical chaos you are experiencing is synonymous with labour, but in reality it is a direct response to fear. Understanding these feelings and learning how to influence the stress cycle will help you avoid reaction. This is why we are going to explore the nature of fear, why it has such power over us today and how it can cause problems during birth.

BIRTH – AN INNER JOURNEY

Being scared during childbirth is not a new phenomenon. Women have probably always been scared at the prospect of giving birth. Fear is a basic and natural instinct, which helps us to survive. But the fear women feel today and the fear women have felt throughout history is wildly different. Since modern western maternity care is one of the safest in the world, we no longer need to worry about illnesses, complications or death during childbirth. Nevertheless, many people working in maternity care today agree that fear of birth is rising amongst women, and that this fear can influence the birthing process in a negative way. This increase of fear has also led to more and more women demanding Caesarean sections, or needing special treatment. Even though women today are more prepared for birth and can expect higher standards of medical care, they are more afraid when it comes to giving birth than ever before. Somewhere in the mix of new technology and the promises of a pain-free existence we have lost something fundamental. Despite all these advances and the ready availability of information many women feel that something is missing – another kind of wisdom, a knowledge that can help them have faith in their own body's ability to prepare for childbirth.

At this given moment of your pregnancy you might think this does not apply to you, and you might not have any fears about the upcoming birth. Some women do not experience any fear during their pregnancy, but find that they unexpectedly become afraid during childbirth. Of course, it is possible that there are some women who are not at all scared before, during or after childbirth. However, I believe most women do experience fear at some point during birth. It is normal. The birthing process is both an extreme and an intense experience; therefore it is only natural that all kinds of feelings and sensations come and go. Fear is just one of these feelings, but if you do not learn to understand what you are feeling, the sensation could escalate and ultimately overwhelm you.

This is why, as a mental preparation, it is very important to understand how fear might affect you, both physically as well as mentally. When you understand the body's reaction to fear and stress, you will be able to apply the four tools presented in this book. These tools will help you to swiftly break or lessen the feeling of fear and the effects it might have on you.

It is like preparing for a hike in the mountains. You assume you will enjoy the trip, that you will be able to complete the journey and that it will give you great joy. You look forward to the feeling after a complete hike of being re-energized and revitalized. Before setting out on the journey you have prepared yourself. You know what to do if there is a storm, and what equipment to bring in case there are unexpected challenges on the way.

You can apply the same mindset when giving birth. The birth is like a hike deep into your inner landscape and this book will serve as your map. You assume this journey is going to strengthen you, that you have the ability to give birth, and that there will be lots of light and joy. But you also need to be prepared in case there are winds and obstacles on the way. You are aware that a storm can be a huge challenge, but you also know that even a great storm will subside eventually – you just need to learn how to weather it. If you get lost, you will, with the right tools and drawing on your inner strength, be able to find your way back to experience the joy of childbirth.

ANCIENT SURVIVAL MECHANISM

We find the answer to the question as to why fear can get in the way of childbirth far back in history. Humans have evolved enormously in a very short time. Today, many of the threatening situations our ancestors met are no longer an issue. Mentally we have mostly learned to adapt to our new situation, but our bodies still carry the reaction patterns of yesterday. Our emotions play an important part as messengers which trigger these chain reactions. Every single emotion has its own unique bodily expression, and its own unique function.

Fear is an alarm signal. It is preparing the body to react when facing potential threats – the fight-or-flight response. The emotion plays the part of a starting engine. It acts as a red alert mechanism preparing the body to meet the challenges and difficult situations ahead. The body will prioritize this red alert system and put the ongoing birth on hold, since this makes most sense for our survival. Stress hormones will rush through the system to give us a boost of energy and sharpen our focus. As our attention increases, vigilance sharpens, the pupils widen, the reproductive system slows down, the muscles get a rush of extra blood and the respiratory system speeds up to oxygenate the muscles. It all makes perfect sense if you look at this from an evolutionary perspective. If our ancient ancestors found themselves in a situation where they were being chased by a bear or any other wild animal, it was important for them to be able to flee in the middle of labour, without giving birth to the baby while on the run.

Problems arise when the threat you are facing is from your own body. In this case what causes the stress reaction does not go away, and the body's response gets in the way of labour. Fear no longer has a purpose. The body does not understand that there is no outer threat. It only responds to the sensation of fear.

Fear has an effect not only on the body, but also on the mind and on the emotions. Tunnel vision sets in, and you can only focus on the danger you are facing. What happens next is that the sensation of pain gets all the attention. Everything but the sensation of pain ceases to exist, as it dominates all other emotions and feelings. If this stress reaction is prolonged, with no time for recovery, it can trigger feelings of hopelessness, and negative emotions might start to take over the birthing experience.

I have seen many labouring women entering negative stress patterns. When I help them to break free from these stress patterns, the experience of childbirth suddenly shifts and they can experience a much wider range of feelings and sensations. They can laugh, sleep, listen to their bodies, cuddle with their partner and so on and so forth. Labour changes from a stressful negative event, to a challenge they can handle.

THE BODY AS A MESSENGER OF MEANING

Why is it that we are afraid of something that is so primal, even though childbirth is safer now than ever before? Today we see labour as a medical matter, and not as something to deepen our emotional intelligence. Our lives revolve more and more on our external surrounding, as opposed to what is happening on the inside. Work, careers and the impossibly difficult puzzle of our lives take most of our attention. The body and its functions have been reduced to something irritating and troublesome. We no longer see the body as a messenger of meaning, or as something important. Today we regard all pain as negative, and we believe we should have the right to live a pain-free life. We do not stop to listen and learn when we feel pain. Many times we see pain as something that gets in our way. It hinders and bothers us in our effort to live our lives the way we want to. When we get a headache, or a muscular pain, or even if our whole body is full of pain, we don't usually stop to ask *why* we are feeling this way. We simply take a pill, or go and see the doctor.

This attitude can create a problem during labour. Suddenly we cannot ignore the signals the body is sending out, and at the same time we can't take all the pain away. We must allow the process to unfold naturally. We are thrown into an extreme physical experience and are expected to know how to deal with it, and how to act. We need to learn how to trust the fact that pain is an important function of childbirth and that our bodies can handle it.

The body is very capable when it comes to giving birth, but you need to understand its functions and learn to read the messages it is giving out. If you fail to read the body's signals, it becomes something alien and dangerous, which in turn creates a separation between you and your own body. The pain and energy of labour might then be experienced as an external power that takes over the body, rendering you more or less helpless. You are reacting to what happens inside of you as if it were an external threat, leaving you feeling scared and triggering the fight-or-flight response. The terror you are feeling tells your body 'you are not allowed to go into labour now, there is a potential threat'. At this point the body puts the brakes on the whole birthing process, potentially causing it to become more drawn out and painful.

Therefore it is necessary to actively build confidence in the body's ability, and to collect all the knowledge needed on how to facilitate the birthing process. You will start to feel a connection to your body if you can understand its signals. Your body will no longer be alien or separate from you. The body and the mind can melt into one in the collective effort – giving birth to a baby!

Listening to your body

You will never be able to predict exactly what is going to happen during labour. Instead it is important to accept everything that occurs, and get to know your thoughts and feelings. Practise listening to what your body is telling you. Notice the changes, such as a growing belly, the baby moving around, the pelvis aching or some other sensation you might experience. The signals might not be that easy to distinguish at first, and might be hard to define, but, with practice, it will get easier and easier to put what you are experiencing into words.

exercise

1. Position yourself comfortably. Turn off all sounds and light a candle. Make sure you are wearing something soft. Close your eyes.
2. Focus on your thoughts. Direct your attention towards what is happening inside of you right now. What thoughts and emotions come up? Notice them for a while. Observe both negative and positive thoughts without judging them. Simply think: 'Here comes a thought or a feeling'.
3. Notice your feelings. What emotions are you filled with right now? Accept all your feelings, even the ones you do not wish to feel: the ones that are hard, difficult or unpleasant. Also welcome the ones that are pleasant, positive, lovely and exciting. Let them come and go without giving in to them. Do not look for reasons as to how or why they are there. Your feelings are not who you are. Simply let them be.
4. Welcome your body's signals. Do the same with your body's sensations. How does the body feel? Tense? Does it hurt? Is it itchy? Relaxed? Do not judge or put any value on what you are experiencing. Simply notice.

▼

5. Now, you are more or less present in the moment. Focus your mind on one sensation: your breathing. Feel your inhalations and exhalations, and how they move through your body. Concentrate on one thing at a time, for example how the stomach moves as you breathe.
6. Let your mind expand and widen. While aware of your breathing, move your attention to your body, from head to toe. While focusing on your breathing and your body, also become aware of your thoughts and emotions. You are your breathing, your body, your emotions and your thoughts combined. The breathing is no longer limited to your respiratory system. You actually breathe with your whole body and mind – it is all one unit.

YOUR EXPERIENCE IS AS IMPORTANT AS MEDICAL SAFETY

Contrary to popular belief, a positive or a negative birth experience is not determined by the kind of pain relief used, where the birth took place, or any complications or external circumstances that might arise. Instead, it is the ability to handle any fears that might arise during labour that will determine how you later judge your experience.

When I first started working as a doula, I thought my work was to help women to have the 'perfect natural birth'. I felt like a failure when complications arose during birth, and I thought the women would be dissatisfied. Instead they seemed very pleased, and felt happy and empowered after giving birth. At first I did not understand why they were so positive. There had been complications! Then I realized that during their entire labour, they had felt as if their feelings were taken seriously, which allowed them to deal better with their fear. That is what determined if they felt positive. This also explained why some women who seemingly had had a very smooth and uncomplicated birthing process would think of it as a negative experience. It was the feeling of fear and anxiety that was negative, and the inability to deal with these feelings. I understood that my task was to protect the experience of labour and not to provide the 'perfect birth'.

The inability to handle feelings of panic and anxiety during labour can also influence a woman's future life and lead to depression, fear of a future pregnancy, low self-confidence, distrust in the body, nightmares, and difficulty bonding with the child. Extreme fear can also directly affect the birthing process, since it activates the stress reactions, which function only to block our bodies. Keeping this in mind, panic and extreme fear should be seen as amongst the most severe complications of labour, and great effort should be put in place to try to avoid these feelings.

Many women feel they lack the inner strategies and tools to meet the challenges and feelings they encounter during labour. Women are often shocked to discover there is little or no help to deal with these issues on the maternity ward. But perhaps it is not up to the maternity ward to provide this type of care. Maybe we have to come to a point where we need to turn inwards in order to find what we are missing. What if the solution is not out there – but inside of us? What if we start to realize that we have all the power and trust we need inside? Our bodies are made to give birth and can show us the way, if we can find a way to listen.

Anita's birth story

I was searching for knowledge, strength, a method and some kind of consolation. Memories of my first son's birth brought feelings of fear, anxiety, pain and humiliation. With a few months to go until my next birth, I realized I did not want to go through the same hell again. Never. I was convinced there had to be another way, with more support and better help to be able to understand how to let go during birth. I got in touch with a midwife, but our conversations did not give me the guidance I needed which I eventually only got from the four tools described in this book. These tools assisted me in giving birth to my second son. It turned out to be a fantastic experience.

I start to feel the early rushes in the evening, but I am able to go to bed with a free and easy mind. I am ready. At night I am awakened by the first contractions and I am able to rely on the relaxation techniques I have been practising for several months. I had forgotten the paralyzing pain, but by focusing on breathing softly and quietly I am still able to doze off in between contractions. I get up around 5 a.m. I am able to meet and welcome the contractions. It is easy to focus and follow along with the help of concentrated breathing (the soft, wonderful breathing). I remind myself not to fight the contractions or to stiffen up in fear of the next contraction.

I keep busy by baking. I meet each irregular rush by closing my eyes and standing upright with my knees slightly bent and my arms hanging loose. I repeat a mantra to myself to make me heavy, heavy, heavy. When my eyebrows start to pull up and tense, my husband firmly strokes my arms and back. His movements are slow and moving downwards.

We have breakfast and the force of my contractions intensifies. It is liberating to end the rushes with a great big sigh to welcome the break.

I have to stand up and receive the contractions now, but I am able to greet them without fear or panic. Nils has to remind me to breathe as the sweat is flowing. We both feel like it is time to leave.

We get to the delivery room and Nils is my primary focus. I have to keep close to him, as he talks me through the contractions, which are now rolling in more and more frequently. He makes my brow relax, my shoulders sink, and he reminds me to breathe quietly. A new awareness of how I am able to work WITH my body rushes over me, and I am not at all scared of the pain.

The waters break with a splash, and the force of the bearing-down contractions makes me lose control. The mantra is gone. The mindfulness of what I am doing is also gone. The only thing that feels real is the touch and the voice of Nils. I have somehow managed to undress and after the other-worldly pain, the baby comes and with him the release, the happiness, the joy and the rush of knowing that this time I have been able to access my inner power and my body in an unbelievably radical way.

BE KIND TO YOURSELF

Before we go on I would like to share an important point with you. This is something you can carry with you. A problem often arises when talking about labour, womanhood, and the fact that you are responsible for yourself. Many women feel they must accomplish something by giving birth or through motherhood. When they don't 'live up to that standard' they tend to feel like failures. It is very important not to look at labour as a performance or as an achievement. I've learnt by experience how impossible it is to know precisely how you are going to react, or what you are going to feel like during labour. Do not judge your feelings as right or wrong. It is not about never feeling fear. The goal is not to give birth completely without doubt. The goal is not to get scared of being scared. What you are trying to do is avoid letting fear take over your birth. Look at fear as a natural part of your labour, and learn how to handle whatever surfaces as and when it happens.

Only look to yourself. Cultivate not only love but also respect for your inner boundaries and whatever obstacles you encounter. Remember that everyone has their own journey, their own unique experience and their own discoveries. You need to feel support and respect, based on the unique person that you are. If you get that, you will automatically be more forgiving towards yourself, and you will also feel empowered by knowing you did your best. Your attitude towards yourself and others will be more forgiving and open-minded if you do not compare your story to those of others. Compare only with yourself and you will find many new ways of growth and opportunity.

Respect yourself and your emotions. Think of fear as an inner emotional challenge that you can take charge over. Avoid identifying yourself as 'the scared one' or 'the brave one'. Instead try to see fear as a natural part of the process, and look at labour as an opportunity to grow according to your own conditions. Do the best that you can. That is enough, because you are the only one who knows what is right or wrong for you. Focus on what you can handle.

Finding the confidence

Your body already knows how to give birth to a baby. Regardless of whether or not you have read or practised specific methods, your baby will be born. The knowledge is already in place and the process is well prepared inside the body. Many generations before you have given birth, and that wisdom is programmed inside of you. The birthing process is a result of hundreds of thousands of years of evolution where Mother Nature, through her fantastic ability to find the optimal solutions, has found this way for us to give life. Everything is thoroughly thought out, down to the very smallest details.

Specific physiological changes need to take place for a child to be born. The cervix area needs to open and expand, and the ligaments need to stretch for the child to be able to squeeze through. These transitions require effort, and women experience them with varying degrees of pain. However, you are fully equipped to handle these changes as long as you allow them to happen. Try the very best you can to trust the body's ability to handle this process, with or without drugs.

Maybe this is where it gets difficult. How? How will you be able to surrender? How can you let the body have access to its innate power? How can you find this confidence?

You want to do the right thing and use the best techniques when you give birth. You want to be well prepared and well read on the subject. You want to feel united as a team with your partner. All of this is important. But what if this is not something you have to teach yourself? What if the preparation you need is to bring out what is already inside of you? You do not have to 'do' anything except try to find a way to fully trust your own ability in an effort to 'surrender' yourself to what is already given and natural.

This is what the four tools are built upon. In the midst of all the methods, all the things you think you need to learn and all the techniques, there is a body; a body that works by a few simple basic physiological principles. If you and your partner know how these basic principles operate, you can easily help the body give birth.

Childbirth is one of the greatest emotional challenges a woman will go through in her lifetime. Your ability to handle emotions and obstacles will be put to the test. During labour, chaos will merge with order, and joy will meet pain. You might experience childbirth as something positive, exciting and challenging, or as something terrifying, chaotic and threatening. All of these sensations can be present during the same birth. Many women are not quite prepared for this emotional paradox. To prepare for this experience you will need to find an inner strength so that you can handle the positive as well as the negative emotions that might emerge during labour.

COPING

Increasing the ability to handle stress is not like learning a new game. We like to see childbirth as an isolated experience, independent from the rest of our lives. However, when we go into labour we bring with us our whole life history. According to Aaron Antonovsky, a professor of medical sociology who has done a lot of research on stress, it is the feeling of *comprehensibility, manageability, and meaningfulness* that determines the ability to handle life. These three components sum up the inner capability to see life as it is, and are crucial when determining how you will handle success as well as setbacks. Childbirth is one of those challenges in life where your attitude to life, and your life experiences, will play an important part. I have been greatly inspired by Antonovsky's three components when writing this book.

Fear and stress arise when you feel you cannot live up to expectations, and when you lack trust in your own ability to handle what is in front of you. In the sixties Richard Lazarus, an American researcher on stress, showed that it is the individual's interpretation of the situation that determines the level of stress he or she is experiencing – not the actual situation itself. This is called coping. Coping means handling and incorporating what inner (thoughts and emotions) and outer (tools, support) resources you have to draw upon when facing stressful situations. To illustrate this I will use a metaphor. A person who meets a wild bear will probably react very differently depending on whether or not he or she is a hunter. A hunter will have the skills to handle the situation. Accordingly, it is not the stress level in itself that determines the stress reaction, but rather the ability and opportunity to influence the situation that is the crucial element.

During childbirth we can translate this into how a woman experiences pain. If she reacts to the labour pains in a negative way, the body will interpret this as a threatening situation which it does not have the ability to deal with, and it will, therefore, get ready for flight. If the woman feels she knows why it hurts, and has faith that she has the tools to influence her level of fear, it will lead to a lower stress level and a diminished feeling of wanting to escape.

My theory is that you need to learn how to cope with what is happening, and not try to take it away. This is very much like going for a run. You know from previous jogs that it will be hard and that you are going to have the urge to walk at some points, but you also know from running before that there will be slopes and wind at your back where you can recover and maybe even enjoy yourself. The most important thing, and what probably keeps you going, is knowing that it will feel much better after you are done. You have developed faith in the process and you have worked out strategies to get to the end of the run. You can use the same thought process when it comes to labour and delivery. The contractions are hills. Some of them are small, but others are big and steep. The pain is the effort that sometimes makes the body ache and throb. As a whole, the experience is like a landscape shifting in colour and shape. The reward is the arrival and the birth of a child – this is what makes the experience meaningful.

COPING/HANDLING

1. COMPREHENSIBILITY

Comprehensibility is an *understanding* of what is happening to you. It means that you are experiencing what happens to you during labour as connected, understandable and significant as opposed to a process which is chaotic, random and illogical. This might involve you gathering knowledge about what happens physically during labour. It also involves you understanding how a labour might bring on many contradictory feelings and emotions and how this is normal. Comprehensibility also entails understanding the specific purpose of pain during labour and how it helps to move the process of birth along.

2. MANAGEABILITY

Manageability implies the trust you have in your own resources when it comes to handling and facing whatever comes your way during labour. *What influence can I have on the experience?* You cannot change the natural process of birth, but you can influence how you handle the rushes by using the four tools.

> ### 3. MEANINGFULNESS
> Meaningfulness involves experiencing all situations, even the difficult ones, as significant and valuable to personal growth. It is worth investing time, involvement and energy in understanding the situation at hand, and recognising that everything has a purpose. For example, during labour it helps to remember that the labour pains are part of the natural process of giving birth. The essential qualities that are necessary when preparing to give birth are *trusting* in your body, and understanding the *meaningfulness* of the birth process. This knowledge will help to protect against fear and stress.

PLACEBO EFFECT

The 'positive placebo' effect is important when it comes to counteracting fear and stress. We all have this fantastic inherent capacity. By believing in a positive outcome the body's own system of power and positive energy is stimulated. The body releases substances to help you – instead of blocking you.

Presently we know a lot about how negative feelings affect our system, but not so much about the effects of positive emotions and how they work. For a long time science has been looking at what makes us unhealthy and sick, both physically and mentally, but not at what makes us thrive. Emotions like happiness, wellbeing, joy, enthusiasm and delight are still relatively unexplored territories. This is about to change. Positive psychology is becoming more and more popular, and it is about focusing on what makes us healthy and well.

Positive emotions kickstart the reward system in the brain, and reduce the stress hormones while lowering the heart rate and relaxing you. This effect is also known as a placebo and has been well known for a long time. It used to be thought of as something negative since doctors would get positive results after having given their patients sugar pills instead of real medicine in clinical trials. Today we understand that this process of self-healing and self-soothing is a very real human response.

I was attending a birth where the woman had previously had a Caesarean section. It had been a negative experience for her and this time she wanted to do things differently. Her mind was set on having a vaginal birth. Her labour started and the days came and went. Even though it took a long time, and there were a few obstacles on the way she never hesitated or changed her mind. She was completely set on giving birth naturally and she did. Importantly, she had no preconceptions as to how long the birth was going to take or what it was going to be like. She was mentally prepared for a second Caesarean, but she knew there was also a good chance that things would turn out the way she wished. After her child was born she was delighted because she felt her dream had come true.

By creating realistic and positive mental pictures of the birth you can get leverage and access your inner powers. The reason I am writing about realistic mental pictures is that unrealistic pictures with expectations that are way over your actual abilities could have the opposite effect. If this particular woman had focused on not taking an epidural, or on the fact that it had to be a quick birth, or that she was going to experience joy all the time, her reaction afterwards could very well have been the opposite. She would probably have ended up being sad, disappointed or angry.

Try to avoid 'locking' your mind on achieving a 'perfect birth' or reaching a specific emotional state. Try not to decide in advance how you are going to feel or react, or how the birth will proceed. Be open to what comes up, because things can happen in many different ways. Use empowering mental pictures where you are prepared to handle anything that happens gracefully and in your own way. This technique will help you prepare to handle the unknown. Dress the pictures in beautiful, positive and light colours.

Empowerment

1. Visualize and write the birth plan as an open-ended event where all emotions are allowed. The goal of this exercise is to be open-minded and be present in what happens. Focus inwards instead of on the outside. Welcome all emotions and feelings, and picture how you are going to get help and support from the people around you. Work with the mindset of love towards yourself. Set a 'non-achieving' intention for the birth and this exercise.

2. Make a staircase of goals. Let the first step be realistic and easy. It can be to handle one contraction at a time, or not to tense up during the rush, or to use the tools to hold fear at bay. The next step might be a little harder. It could be the decision as to whether or not to use an epidural or another form of pain relief. This may lead to you being able to take one thing at a time and to get the satisfaction of managing the first step before going on to the next.

TRUST

The trust I will talk about in this chapter is the feeling of *innate trust*. It is very important and will give you a lot of support during labour. Innate trust is having confidence in the fact that things will work out fine, and that there is something that provides support regardless of whether or not you have any religious faith. Trust will shelter you from fear, stress and anxiety. You can lean on it in times of weakness and it is a source of strength. Innate trust is there as a foundation for you when dealing with what life throws at you. Negative feelings and thoughts can grow and take over where there is no trust.

People today place a great trust in society and the things around them, but not so much so when considering their own body. The self-healing aspects of the human body are overlooked and instead we put a lot of faith in medical science. The feeling of taking part and being included in the birth disappears when the woman completely gives herself over to hospital care in the belief that they can handle the birth for her. Hospitals are partly to blame for this attitude since many things in that environment, and the routines surrounding childbirth, signal danger and fear. Childbirth needs to be seen both by the hospital and by women as something natural and not as a potential danger so that we are better able to access our innate trust.

To protect against fear and stress during labour it is necessary to build a foundation of trust. The ability to have this trust is dependent on the woman's life history, but I think this trust is innate and that it can be awakened regardless of what has happened in the past. There are probably several things in everyday life that might be risky, but that we still have faith and trust in. We have faith and trust every time we sit down in an aeroplane or start the car or make important decisions. All of these things would be very difficult if we felt any anxiety or worry.

It is not important exactly who or what you put your faith or trust in. You might feel trust in your body or in the knowledge it contains. You might put your faith in the hospital and the competence of the staff, in your partner or your doula or even in the child. All these factors play an important part when it comes to letting go and letting the body give birth. Look at it as an active choice to build up positive role models, and faith and trust in the body.

exercise

Preparing for a confident birth: Trust

- Trust in your body's ability to give birth.
- Remember that childbirth is a natural process.
- Trust in the self-healing aspects of the human body.
- Trust in the four tools to help you through the birth.
- Put your faith in your partner, your doula or the hospital staff who are there to support you and will look after you, even when you feel scared.

MEANINGFULNESS

Meaningfulness and inherent trust are closely related to one another. Both of these feelings trigger the placebo effect whereby positive expectations counteract the pain. By understanding what is happening you can protect yourself from the negative emotions that can lead to fear. By finding a deeper meaning, birth becomes a meaningful event in itself.

The meaning of childbirth is individual and as complex as each individual life. One woman found her trust when, after 24 hours of unsuccessful inductions, she asked for a Caesarean section. By making this decision, she grew and felt empowered and thought of childbirth as a positive event. Another woman got a similar feeling when she was able to give birth without using pain medication with the help of her husband, doula and midwife. This was a source of strength for her for many years afterwards. A third woman drew her strength from the fact that she dared to give birth at all, using all the drugs and help she could get. After this she felt she could face other difficult areas in her life. What all these women have in common is that they all decided to face their own fears and not let them take over and govern them. All three women shared the same faith and trust in the meaning of the birth process. This is a meaning you have the power to create for yourself.

THE BODY'S YES AND NO

The purpose of the four tools is to counteract the body's negative stress reaction by activating the opposite system. The opposite of stress is safety, or the 'peace and calm system'. The stress reaction can be seen as a 'no'. The body receives information about a possible danger ahead and locks down to work against the birth. However, the 'peace and calm system' can be seen as a 'yes' from the body since its primary message is safety and the reassurance that things are the way they are supposed to be.

The peace and calm system belongs to the parasympathetic nervous system, while the stress reaction belongs to the sympathetic nervous system. Together they make up the autonomic nervous system. Both of these components are equally important, and certain activations of the stress system during labour can be positive. It is the negative stress, connected to fear, that can influence the birth in an adverse way. The most important substance of the peace and calm system is the hormone oxytocin. Oxytocin releases a sort of anti-stress function via the endorphin system – the body's most important system when it comes to pain relief. Oxytocin is released in response to touch and warmth and induces feeling of security and calmness. But, it is also affected by our thoughts and emotions and has a clear anxiety-prohibiting effect. It also has a pain-relieving quality. The pain is registered, but is not felt so strongly and is not so threatening. Professor Kerstin Uvnäs Moberg has conducted extensive research into this crucial and magical hormone in her book *The Oxytocin Factor*.

Oxytocin is the hormone which plays an important role in breastfeeding and in the work of contractions. It is fascinating that the body has chosen oxytocin, which is connected to pleasure and security, as the key hormone during childbirth. Labour is not what most people think of as pleasure. However, it has to do with the body's 'yes' and 'no'. We are meant to give birth in safety and confidence, away from danger.

The four tools will help you to counteract the emotions that inhibit the birth process and give you the confidence to find your own way. Each of the tools you will learn in the following chapter will help you to open up the inner capacity of your body, and enable you to find your own way to give birth. They will not necessarily take the pain away or make the process of giving birth 'easy', but they will help you to find a way to work with your body and not against it.

PAIN MEDICATION

Many people ask if pain medication is not enough when dealing with pain. I am often asked if I am for or against drugs during labour. Do I think it is good or bad, natural or unnatural? I have been present at births taking place at hospitals and in private homes. I have been present at births both with and without analgesia, as well as Caesarean births. Some births have had a lot of complications while many, many births have had no complications at all. What I have learned from all these births and after all these years as a doula is that it is not the exterior circumstances that determine if the birth ends up being a positive or negative experience, but the inner circumstances.

The questions about pros and cons when it comes to pain medications are too complex and nuanced to cover in this book and there are no easy answers. All medical interventions can have side-effects, and it is important to know about them so that they are not seen as an easy way out. One woman I assisted as a doula described the decision as to whether or not to have an epidural as swapping one bad thing for another. At the end it was hard to know which one was worse.

Sometimes the pros outweigh the cons when it comes to using pain relief during labour since not all natural births are easy or uncomplicated. What is important when making the decision is that you do not decide to use drugs thinking that they will eliminate all pain, or because you are afraid. Scientific research points to many women using pain relief because of fear. The same research showed that these women found labour to be a negative and frightening experience, despite the use of a pain-killing medicine.

From this we can conclude that pain relief does not have an effect on these feelings. Medications for pain relief will help take the edge off the pain if it gets overwhelming. They can also be used as a tool to make the labour process manageable in some cases. However, other strategies will need to be adopted to handle your emotions during labour, which might be more subtle and less specific than what you are used to. But these are the strategies that will help you get through the process, and they are essential when it comes to determining how you end up feeling about the birth. It is how you *experience* the birth, not how it actually is, that either strengthens you, or gets you down. How you personally experience the birth will also determine how you feel about giving birth again in the future. *Coping* is therefore a more important factor than analgesia when it comes to childbirth.

Summary

Our bodies are designed for the physical experience of childbirth. The challenge is to allow it to happen organically.

- Fear is a normal and natural emotion. It is there to protect you against dangers.
- The body reacts to the emotion of fear by preparing to deal with a hostile situation. You are supposed to re-evaluate the situation you are facing. If there is no threat, all the alarm systems in your body will turn off and everything will return to normal.
- Problems occur when the danger or the fear you are feeling is inside your own body. What could be seen as threatening is not disappearing and the stress reactions are prolonged, causing you harm in the long run.
- To avoid this you have to realize it is the fear not the pain that breaks you down. If you can come to an understanding of how the body reacts to positive as well as negative emotions, you can enhance the positive and break or reduce the negative effects.
- It is your perception of fear and pain that determines the stress reaction. This is called coping. If you recognize fear you will also know how to deal with it and, in the end, lessen the stress reaction.
- Use the power of positive energy to minimize the momentum of fearful emotions. If you have confidence in your ability to give birth and believe in the fact that there is a meaning to whatever you are going through, everything will work out fine and you

can free up your body's ability to heal. You will walk out of the experience of childbirth a stronger woman.

- Pain serves a purpose. To lessen the power of fear you need to understand what that purpose is. During the contractions, you will utilize the four tools, described later in this book. Learn to understand why and how the contractions work.

Accept your fear. Learn to live with it, but find a way of facing up to it and dealing with it. Look at fear as a natural aspect of childbirth, but dare to go against your first impulse of running away, and allow yourself to go with the flow.

The birth

We now have the knowledge of how stress and fear can affect a woman's body and mind. We also have more tools and inner strategies to face and handle the positive as well as the negative emotions that might emerge during labour. Now we will look at the natural and healthy birth process and how the body is made for the physical changes that will occur. But we will also look at the things that can cause fear or confusion, even if they are natural, so that you can better differentiate between the natural process and the reactions to fear.

Pain connected to labour often triggers fear, which in turn will start stress reactions. This is often a result of the woman not understanding the purpose of pain. It only feels destructive and meaningless. The pain is, in this case, nothing but an unpleasant sensation that keeps growing and growing. After an energetic workout you might experience muscle pain. It can be quite painful at times, but it never scares you because you know it is a sign of you getting stronger. If that same sensation were to hit you all of a sudden while you are relaxing on the sofa it might scare you since you would not know why you were in such pain. Therefore you need to understand that the pain is a messenger which updates you on the physical changes that take place during labour. This knowledge will lessen the feeling of being overtaken by pain without any ability to influence the situation. You will be able to create meaningful mental pictures by making sense of the contractions. This will make the contractions more understandable and concrete. Childbirth is no longer a threat, but rather a physically demanding job for which you have all the necessary tools at your disposal.

THE PERFECT BODY

I have written this book with normal and healthy childbirth in mind. If you have any specific worries or concerns that scare you, you could of course look into those areas in greater detail. If something unexpected or out of the ordinary occurs during labour, my experience is that the staff will let you know what is happening and what they are going to do about it. Births taking place in hospitals, as well as in private homes, are pretty safe today. This is thanks to the extensive knowledge and understanding of midwives and obstetricians, both on how to prevent and how to foresee possible complications. We should not forget what a marvellous construction the body is. It is a place where hundreds of functions interplay seamlessly every day.

THE FEMALE BODY

Before moving on, I would like to take a closer look at the female body. I will explain some important concepts that are closely linked to labour. You will get a picture of how amazing your body is and how everything is prepared and arranged.

The UTERUS is a pear-shaped sleek muscle with a space in the middle. This is the space in which the baby will grow for the next nine months. The uterus of a woman before conception is small like a pear and hidden behind the pubic bone. It will expand when the baby grows and at the end of the pregnancy it will have reached all the way up to your lower ribcage. You cannot control this muscle by will. It is, however, connected to your sympathetic nervous system which is very sensitive to fear and negative emotions.

CERVICAL MUSCLE This is the way in or out of the uterus, depending on which perspective you are taking. The cervix connects the uterus to the vagina. At the beginning of labour the cervical muscle is around four centimetres in length, but it shortens and softens as labour progresses. What is left at the end of this process is an opening called the mouth of the womb, or the cervix. This ring-shaped muscle widens during each contraction until it reaches ten centimetres in diameter.

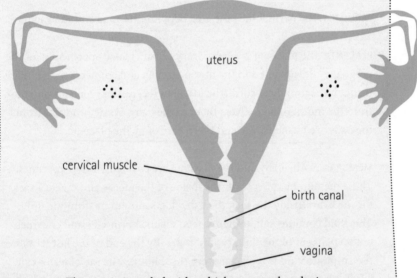

uterus

cervical muscle

birth canal

vagina

MUCUS PLUG The cervix is sealed with a thick mucus plug during pregnancy. The mucus plug protects the entrance to the uterus.

BIRTH CANAL The birth canal is the tunnel connecting the uterus to the vagina. It is a mucus membrane, able to expand and tighten like an accordion, diagonally as well as vertically.

VAGINA The vagina consists of two inner labia. Because of their vertical shape they are able to fit around the baby's head as it pushes through.

PELVIC FLOOR The pelvic floor is the muscular base of the abdomen and is attached to the pelvis. It supports and holds up the inner organs. You can feel these muscles if you squeeze your anus and your sex organs. The pelvic floor will help you to push the baby out.

PERINEUM The perineum is the area between the anus and the vagina.

PLACENTA The placenta is a temporary organ created specifically for the pregnancy. It is planted in the uterine lining, and connects to the infant through the umbilical cord. The placenta receives oxygen and nutrition from the mother and delivers them to the baby. Waste products from the baby are flushed away and taken care of by the placenta.

MEMBRANES The baby and the placenta are covered with membranes. These membranes also cover the inside of the uterus and create a sack for the baby. Inside the sack the baby floats around in amniotic fluid. This fluid contains salt, proteins, fats, sugars, hormones and enzymes, but 95 per cent of the fluid is pure water. By the end of the last trimester the amniotic fluid is replaced every three hours. The sac of water can break at any time during labour, but sometimes the baby is born with the amniotic sac intact. When this happens people say the baby is 'born with a caul' or 'born to succeed'.

OXYTOCIN This hormone is also referred to as the 'love hormone' or the 'feel-good hormone'. Oxytocin is produced when you feel safe, relaxed, secure and peaceful. It is involved in starting the contractions.

COMMON WORRIES BEFORE LABOUR

Fear of the unknown is a normal human reaction, and it is quite normal to be worried about giving birth. You will have many questions which you will want to answer to help you to understand the challenge ahead. Will I be able to handle the birth? Will my body be able to cope? The questions can also be spiritual or existential. What is the purpose of pain? You might not even know specifically why you are anxious, because the worry is more about facing something you have always heard is painful.

To be able to process these thoughts and emotions a woman needs to be seen, respected and listened to. Her feelings should be taken seriously, however irrational they might appear. She needs to accept and respect all emotions, but be mindful and work actively to process them so that they do not overwhelm her. From science we know that women who expect a negative birth experience, will evaluate their own childbirth as negative after delivery. It can be a self-fulfilling prophecy, where the negative energies release blocking substances that will work against the body. This reaction is called nocebo, or the negative expectation effect; it is the opposite of the positive expectation effect, or placebo, I talked about earlier.

You do not have to eradicate every ounce of fear to prevent this, but you need to distance yourself from the fear. You can choose not to react to the fear, and not let it take over. Make a decision beforehand to have as a goal to learn to deal with fear, rather than trying to eradicate it. We are going to take a closer look at common sources of worries. If you have the chance to reflect on your worries beforehand, you will have a more realistic and deeper understanding of them.

TWO TYPES OF WORRIES

After many years working on the maternity ward, I feel I can distinguish two different kinds of fear in labour. The first group consists of women who have either been close to someone who has had a traumatic birth experience or they themselves have first-hand experience of a difficult birth. It can involve complications, feelings of abandonment or of being lost. This fear is always connected to the actual situation. The second group includes women who have deep, unresolved issues from earlier events in their lives. Women in the first group can be helped by taking specific steps to prevent the trauma from recurring. The second group can partly be helped by this approach, but it is usually not enough. They need assistance in getting an understanding of the underlying cause of their fear.

I was hired to be a doula for a woman who had a very bad relationship with her mother. Her mother was a drug addict and had not been able to give her daughter a basic sense of security. The woman and her partner hired me because of her fear of birth. We worked on this fear throughout her pregnancy. During one of our talks I asked if she had any fears about becoming a mother. She reflected on this and realized she was afraid to deliver her baby. What if she could not love a child? What if she were to harm her baby emotionally, just like she had been hurt? She was given the space to articulate her thoughts, and through the conversation she could see how she already was a good mother by daring to talk about these issues, and being aware of them. She felt hope returning and was looking forward to meeting her child. This made her fear of delivery more or less vanish. One month later she gave birth to a son and everything went well.

It is not necessary to go through extensive therapy to be able to handle fear. The simple act of trying to look at the problem from several different angles can help to articulate the fears and overcome the emotional hurdles. The difficult things in life can be transformed into an enormous strength.

PREVIOUS NEGATIVE BIRTH EXPERIENCE

The fear that occurs after a previous negative birth experience is often connected to an underlying distrust, either of the healthcare system, of one's partner, or of one's own body. The fear itself is usually connected to the previous experience. The woman might have had expectations or thoughts on how it was going to be. When the labour did not happen as planned she was left feeling disappointed. Another scenario is that the woman might have looked forward fearlessly to the birth, only to discover that it was not at all what she had expected. The force and pain might have been stronger and harder to handle than she had imagined. Alternatively, the pain might not have been the problem but she was left feeling alone and vulnerable.

To be able to process the experience the woman needs to be allowed to talk about it. The conflict may be in the fact that everything went well from a medical point of view but not at all well from an emotional perspective. She might think it is taboo to discuss her feelings, or she might not even be aware of this inner turmoil. Much energy is wasted, and the event is not being dealt with. Sometimes the woman does not know who is to blame, but is just left with a feeling that she did not get what she needed, and she wanted something that the healthcare system could not offer.

She needs to learn from the experience, as it will help her to understand what she needs to do differently to prepare for the upcoming birth. It is possible to heal the wounds from past experiences with the help of a new birth, and I have been lucky to witness this amazing transformation many times. Memories of the new experience act like a veil, covering the old wounds and replacing them with positive emotions.

Preparing for a confident birth:
Reduce the fear caused by a previous negative birth experience
- Educate yourself so that you know what emotions and feelings to expect.
- Try using specific techniques to handle your emotions.
- Find supportive people who will empower you and give you a sense of security.

NEGATIVE INFLUENCES FROM OTHERS

Fear can come from the inside or from the outside. Some people have an almost pathological need to tell horrific birth stories as soon as they spot a pregnant woman. It is not okay to do so! And you have the right to put your foot down. To protect yourself you need to kindly, but firmly indicate that you do not need to hear the story that person wants to tell you. Instead, try talking to people who will bring out the positive, empowering images of birth. Simply cut out the negative as much as possible.

Too much information about what can go wrong during pregnancy and delivery can create anxiety and fear. Ask yourself if it is really necessary to know everything that could possibly go wrong. When you get in your car you do not automatically think of the accidents you might get into or of all the horrible injuries those accidents might involve. Rather than anticipating events that will possibly never happen you should instead put your faith in the people around you, safe in the knowledge that they will give you all the help they can in the unlikely event that anything should go wrong.

Sometimes I get criticized when I compare giving birth to driving a car. I am aware that they are not directly comparable. However, it can help to put things into perspective if you think about how impossible it would be to drive if you were to focus on all the things that could go wrong. I do not suggest you should repress your feelings. Talk about your fears, but do not focus on them all the time. You will then have the opportunity to find out if other people share your worries, and it will help you to understand why you are so concerned.

FEAR OF NOT HAVING SUPPORT

Support and security have an enormous influence on negative emotions and stress reactions. Many women realize they will need a lot of support during childbirth. It is important to be seen and respected and not to be alone while giving birth.

Take your emotions seriously. Talk to your partner about what is important to you. Ask him to be honest about his feelings. It is a new situation for both of you. If your partner is as insecure as you are, it is time to look at alternatives. Maybe you can get the help of a doula, a friend or your mother. Women's views of their relationship to their partner have proven to increase when an extra person is present during labour. If you feel you did not get sufficient support from your partner you might feel hurt and deserted. It can take a while to rebuild that trust. If all the responsibility does not fall on your partner, the extra support can actually help him to strengthen his role. Be clear about what sort of assistance you need when you communicate with the hospital staff. You might want them to praise you, be close to you, to use certain words or to do something entirely different. Many women do not do this, for fear of being 'difficult', but it is very valuable information for the staff since they do not know you.

Your support person also needs information on how to be a better assistant. The support person is often expected to automatically know how to support a woman in childbirth. Daily life is very different from childbirth and it is unfair to expect the support person to know what you need in this situation. At the end of the book I have included a chapter aimed at the support person.

Preparing for a confident birth:
Reduce the fear of not receiving sufficient support
- Talk about what kind of assistance you need.
- Be honest.
- Clearly communicate your needs to the staff.

Elin's birth story

After delivering my first baby I was not feeling at all well. I had a great need to process everything, but the feeling of disappointment would not lose its grip. I had been so prepared, charged, and rested, and I had a high threshold for pain. In spite of all this I ended up with medical procedures, an episiotomy, vacuum extractors and a deep concern for the baby. Immediately afterwards I was in pain from the stitches, and had a hard time bonding with my baby. All I could think about was the 36-hour-long birth process and everything that had happened during that time.

Before birth number two, I tried not to make the same mistake of

connecting all my self-esteem to how I experienced the birth. But I knew
I was in great need of a positive birth experience to be able to handle an
infant and a three year old. I contacted a doula to increase my chances of
having the kind of birth I wanted, and to feel like I had done what I could.
It was a relief to have someone beside me who knew what I wanted and
who could support me when things got hard. Just as before, I would have
preferred not to have any medical pain-relief, and perhaps only laughing
gas. I just wanted to know how much pain nature intended me to feel,
and I wanted to do everything in my power to avoid complications for
my baby. I was given an intravenous injection during my first delivery,
on the assumption I was too tired, and to be able to receive contraction
stimulation medicine. This may have been a good decision, or maybe the
baby would have felt better if I had not been stressed from the beginning.
This I will never know.

My over-riding concern this time was that I would get depressed after
yet another disappointing delivery. I was also worried I would be taken by
surprise by the pain, since I had hardly experienced any pain last time. I
spoke to my doulas about my experiences and I felt I moved a little further
in the process. I had found women who understood how I had felt cheated
by my experience, and how I had a lack of faith in my body. I decided not
to flee, but to stay, relax and let go.

After two false alarms with Braxton Hicks contractions, I was happy
when it seemed like labour had started for real – and on the right day
as well. The contractions came regularly, and we were admitted at 10.35
pm on the Sunday night. At the hospital everything took a turn for the
worse and got scary and uncomfortable. I no longer wanted to give birth.
I wished I could take a pill to stop the process. The examination showed
I was only three centimetres dilated and the cervix was intact. This left

me with a heavy feeling. Maybe my body could not do this after all? Furthermore, my baby's head was turned the wrong way, just like my first. This was not a good start and I was overwhelmed by the same old feelings. I hesitated to call my doula. I thought I could not ask her to be at the hospital for 20 hours, and it would be better to save her for a real crisis. I ended up calling her in after all, since I felt so scared and lonely at the hospital. With my partner, I managed to walk a few rounds in the hospital hallway before she showed up. The contractions came frequently and it felt good to know my doula and my partner could take it in turns to massage me.

During the contractions I worked consciously to stop ending up in the fight-or-flight behaviour. I struggled to keep my feet firmly on the ground and to keep my face relaxed. It was impossible to keep my shoulders and my back relaxed. I received help from my support people who gave me a very helpful massage. No panicky feelings and the contractions kept coming. I was happy the contractions came as closely as they did, so that they would not send me home after all. I had no other pain relief in mind, other than my TENS-machine that was running at half speed. I had not thought about laughing gas. If a midwife had suggested gas I would probably have lost my focus and confidence, which in turn might have made me more aware of the difficulties and the pain. Besides, I had all night in front of me so I thought it was best to hold fire. It was somewhat frightening how hard it was already. Maybe I would not be able to get through it without pain-killers if it went on for too long. It was not exactly painful, but rather a scary sense of pressure bearing down on me. 'Do not be scared', I kept repeating to myself. 'It is just an uncomfortable sensation. It is part of the process.' Time went fast. Swish, and two hours had passed since we came in.

At 1.15 am the midwife thought I looked a little sweaty. She wanted to see if things had been moving along. I felt so happy when she said I was dilated a full ten centimetres and the baby was on its way! No wonder I had felt pressure. I had a lot of strength left and I dared to give birth. After making sure it was okay I put all my strength into the pushing, and my baby son emerged after three contractions.

The two tiny stitches did not even hurt and I had a completely different start when I became a mother of two. My legs shook violently, but it was mostly comically. I did not want to rest. I was savouring my birth experience and treated myself to a couple of aspirin to combat the afterpains.

Afterpain is normal and is just the body's way of adjusting to the change after the baby is born. Nevertheless it can be uncomfortable and especially if you are a multiparous woman. Use a warm beanbag or hot water bottle to help you relax while the body does its job restoring.

One of my first thoughts right afterwards was how unbelievably strong I had been during my first birth which had been so much harder. Why had I walked around feeling like a failure, when in fact it had been a great achievement?

Before my second birth I had been prepared to accept that I would have to live my life with feelings of failure. Now, I am grateful for the humbleness I have received. The most important support this time came from my doula, who shared her belief in my body and its ability to give birth. When these doubts were gone I dared to stay put and give birth my way.

Contractions

The contractions are the most central part of the birth. They help to move the process along, whatever phase the labour happens to be in. This is also when you will experience the most pain, since most of the body's work happens during the contractions. In between contractions you will probably not feel any pain at all. The word contraction is used as an overall term to describe the enormous muscular work done by the uterine muscles during all phases of labour. Contractions occur when the uterus squeezes tightly either to open the cervix, or to push the baby out towards the opening of the vagina.

The entire contraction can be looked upon as an ocean wave, where all the muscle threads of the uterus tighten and relax during approximately 60 seconds.

1. The motion of the wave begins when the upper part of the uterus tightens to press the baby down towards the opening of the cervix. The force spreads down to make the cervix open up even more. It takes approximately 30 seconds for this part of the contraction to reach its peak. This is when the contraction is the most intense.
2. During the next 30 seconds the muscle threads will gradually relax and the pain will subside.
3. Picture the movement like the action of wringing and then untwisting a dishcloth.

The goal of the contraction is to open the cervix, which is placed approximately ten centimetres from the opening of the vagina at the beginning of the birth canal. The cervix has to widen from zero to ten centimetres during labour so that it can allow the baby to pass through the birth canal. After that the pushing contractions take over.

The pain you might experience during labour is caused by the cervix dilating. Numerous pain receptors are situated around the cervical opening. This is the way the body is designed, and it works because you are constantly reminded of the progress of labour.

You might experience great pain during a contraction and still see no visual result. Remember that your body is working to bring you closer to the goal even if you are not 'opening up' during every single contraction.

1. Think of the opening of the cervix rather like trying to put a polo-neck sweater over a baby's head. The force of the contractions pulls the sweater over the baby's head little by little.
2. The cervical opening is like a small ring, noticeable to the touch. The diameter of the ring expands as the sweater is pulled over the head of the baby, until the eyes of the baby are lined up at the opening. The maximum capacity of the ring is reached at ten centimetres in diameter.

The length of the contractions varies depending on which stage of the birthing process the woman is in. The beginning of labour is like a time to warm up and the contractions might last anywhere from 15 to 45 seconds. When the labour is more established the contractions become stronger and longer. They all last for around the same amount of time, and are anywhere between 60 and 90 seconds long.

RHYTHM OF CONTRACTIONS

Contractions have a rhythm, which is created by the length of the rushes and the breaks in between. The contractions are like waves on the ocean, creating a balance between hard work and rest. The rhythm is not new, or foreign to your body. Rather, it is reminiscent of the movement of your breathing, the beating of the heart, or your muscles tightening and then relaxing.

This built-in rhythm is a prerequisite for you to make it through the whole process. The contractions are there to create a balance between hard work and rest. Nature has designed contractions as close to perfection as possible. Contractions are not a destructive pain that does not ease off. Instead of one long contraction that would result in the woman becoming exhausted, the contractions are broken into intervals. An active contraction lasting for approximately 60 seconds is followed by a break that could last for hours in the early stages of labour, and just a few seconds at the end of the process. However, if the level of stress hormones is high during labour, the woman could lose the connection with this rhythm. If she does, she might experience the contractions as bottomless or as one long endless contraction.

The four tools in this book will help you to reduce the stress and to use the breaks between the rushes to rest and to gather strength. This is important since many women find that lack of sleep is a major obstacle. By making good use of the breaks you will be able to flow with the body in its rhythm, no matter how long labour lasts.

The early phases of the birth process can seem erratic. One break might be a few minutes long, only to be followed by another much longer break. Once you have entered the second stage (the opening phase), your contractions become more regular.

PAIN DURING CONTRACTIONS

Pain during childbirth is a symbol of the unknown. It's what your intellect cannot grasp and understand. To be faced with the unknown naturally creates respect and wonder in you. Will I be able to handle this? Will I get scared? This is not unusual, since pain during childbirth can be one of the strongest pains a person will ever experience. This does not automatically make the pain destructive or negative. Pain during childbirth is very different from the pain caused by an injury or trauma, and does not have to involve suffering. Destructive pain signals injury, while pain during labour tells the story of physical transformations in your body. Pain caused by an injury does not give you intermissions where you can rest and recover. In contrast, the breaks between contractions in normal childbirth are times when you can relax and recoup your energy.

Many women describe the pain during labour as being as intense as any destructive pain. They are talking about the peak of the contraction, when the pain is at its most acute state. There are variations in pain during a single contraction. It is like a wave, where the middle of the contraction is the peak. The beginning and the end are like hallways in and out of pain. The strongest part of the contraction can be as acute as destructive pain, but the difference is that it is only acute for a limited time, and you get time to recover when it is over. You will not pass out from pain during a regular birth, as you might from destructive pain. Pain is a warning signal but that is only one of its many functions. Pain can be linked to organic functions signalling a forthcoming event. Pain during labour is the same as the growing pains experienced by a child, the pain of a tooth pushing through the gums, or the cramps felt when the egg and mucus membrane are forced out during menstruation. Obviously it can be an extremely powerful sensation, but that still does not make it negative. However powerful the pain might be, it maintains its positive function.

It is the emotional charge that determines if the pain is perceived as positive or negative. Pain alone is not usually the cause of negativity during labour. Instead, it is the negative emotions connected to the pain that are traumatic. The woman might feel alone, scared, imprisoned or unable to make a move. These feelings create suffering. Nevertheless, it is possible to be in pain without suffering, and to suffer without being in pain. However, if you have a solid base of inner trust, a support system surrounding you, and the means to handle whatever comes to you, the pain does not have to come with suffering. The pain can simply be reduced to a sensation you must endure.

A woman I was assisting suddenly burst into laughter when the pain got unbearable. At first I thought she was crying, but then I realized her tears came from laughter. Between contractions she kept saying how stupid women must be to ever want to do something as idiotic as giving birth. The laughter became a release and her system flooded with endorphins and oxytocin, giving her the distance she needed not to get lost in suffering. You obviously do not have to laugh your way through childbirth, but looking at pain as something natural can be liberating and can help to ease the anxiety and stress of labour.

Preparing for a confident birth: Reduce the fear of pain
- Educate yourself about what causes pain during childbirth.
- Limit the image of pain to the time of the contraction or about 60 seconds.
- Make sure you have sufficient support when labour is at its most intense.

exercise

LETTING GO

Letting go and allowing the natural birth process to happened during the contractions is very important during labour. At the same time this can also very scary and many women get trapped in trying to control the process. Many women are scared of losing control when giving birth. Losing control can be frightening, especially if it is connected to stress and fear. Giving birth can involve you losing control over your body to some extent. For some women, this is in great contrast to their everyday lives.

There is positive as well as negative control. Trusting your body, feeling participatory and in command of your inner tools is control in a positive way. With a foundation of positive control you will feel in command of the things you can influence or steer. You will not be able to control the birth process, but you can work actively at handling fear and stress. Trying to control what is outside of your reach, such as pain, the physical events of the birth or the time it takes to give birth, is negative.

Ask yourself if it is always negative to lose control. Letting go of control, as opposed to losing control, is a positive action. The techniques described in this book will show you how to relinquish control, and allow the birth to proceed. *Letting go* and *surrendering* are closely related. A sense of trust and security is essential to be able to *surrender* to something.

Sexuality is an example of this. You need to be able to partially let go and lose control to be able to feel pleasure and reach an orgasm. Birth is also a situation where complicated physical and mental functions need to interplay, even though it is not quite the same as sex. Therefore, it might be a good preparation to reflect over what circumstances you need to allow you to surrender to a bodily experience. What should the atmosphere around you be like?

Preparing for a confident birth:
Reduce the fear of losing control

- Define what losing control means to you.
- Plan in advance the help you would like to receive in the event you get stuck in these emotions.
- Articulate ways in which losing control could be positive for you.

exercise

LENGTH OF BIRTH

The goal is to manage the labour by handling one contraction at a time and taking advantage of the rest in between. Nevertheless the length of the whole process can be of concern, both if it's very long or so fast that there is no time to get to the hospital.

Many women wonder how they will manage to get through a prolonged labour, with hours upon hours of pain. A process like that will obviously tire you, physically as well as mentally. But it is important to take the opportunity to rest whenever possible, whether the labour lasts for just a few hours or four consecutive days. There is always a break between the rushes, and it is sometimes even possible to fall asleep during labour. Many things can prevent a woman from using these breaks to their best advantage, such as false expectations, feelings of excitement, stress reactions or simply a lack of insight on how to recover. Often women know that they should try to relax, rest and sleep when labour starts, but it can feel impossible to do so. The art of knowing how to relax can be one of the most crucial preparations for the birth and can make the difference between a positive and a negative birth experience. No techniques in the world will be of any help to you if your mental powers are exhausted. You will learn more about how you can sleep and rest during labour in the next section.

The other side of the coin is if the birth happens too quickly, though this is uncommon in first-time mothers. A very fast delivery is mostly an emotional problem, since the pain is concentrated and there are no breaks. There might not be time to understand what is going on, which can be very stressful. If you do not get scared you will find the strength to turn your gaze inwards and to get in touch with what is happening. Most of the time the body works perfectly and there is seldom anything wrong. If you feel you won't make it to the hospital or birthing centre you might do best to stay where you are, in the car or at home, to get as good a birth experience as possible. Your partner can talk to the midwife or obstetrician on the telephone.

If you are worried, talk to your midwife and make a plan for how you are going to deal with a fast childbirth. It is better to be prepared, than to worry about something you cannot control.

It is important not to get fixated on exactly how things will play out in any of the above scenarios. Stay focused on what is actually happening and make sure you have the knowledge to handle the contractions.

exercise

Preparing for a confident birth:
Reduce the fear of a long or quick birth
- Shift the adrenaline gear down so that you can recoup your energy whenever you have the chance.
- Do not decide beforehand how long you think the birth is going to take.
- Learn what you need to know to be prepared for a quick birth.

Björk's birth story

Early Saturday morning I felt a dull pain. Took a warm bath. Called the hospital to warn them. However, the contractions never got regular and had vanished by lunchtime. Sunday morning I once again had a dull aching sensation, but only a few real contractions. The whole family laid down for a nap. Everyone except me fell asleep. The contractions start at ten to four and this time they are regular, three in ten minutes.

We leave for the hospital, which is an hour and a half away. I am sitting deeply focused in our little car. Thinking 'down', 'let go'. I breathe softly, calmly, and I sigh. The contractions grow more and more powerful and I think to myself 'Yeees, we are doing beautifully', my child and I. Feel a deep and sincere collaboration with the baby in my belly. Everything outside, the sun, the people and the cars, my husband's excitement, gets very little of my attention. I dive deeper and deeper into the depth of myself (the universe). When I come up to the surface, words like 'we will make it', 'calm and powerful', and 'love' emerge as soon as I start tensing up.

I ask my husband if he is calm. Then I ask him to stop at an empty layby. I bring a towel and start walking towards the forest. It seems to summon me. I have barely taken my trousers off as the first strong pushing contraction washes over me. I am holding my hands above my baby's head. I am kneeling down, focusing my eyes on an insect. My husband, on the phone, comes running. I yell: 'pull it out'. My husband wonders how, but the baby comes out with a splash and a beautiful scream (on the second push). He throws the phone away and catches the baby.

We are wrapped in damp towels, still linked to each other by the umbilical cord. Above, the sun is gleaming through the leaves. We are covered in bark and leaves. The child, still genderless to us, looks at the world with big, dark, curious eyes. Soon the ambulance arrives and inside we look and see, it's a girl.

The stages of labour

An understanding of the normal birth process can help a woman to recognise the purpose of pain and make it easier for her to react to overcome stress and fear. Giving birth and being born are both physiological and psychological events, yet childbirth today is often reduced to a medical procedure, and treated in the same way as surgery on the physical body. But childbirth is much more than a physical process, and the woman's feelings, thoughts and emotions all have a part to play. Therefore we need to look at childbirth in more holistic terms, because emotions very much contribute to the medical and physical process.

THE STAGES OF LABOUR

1. The *first stage* of labour, also called the latent phase, is when the cervix ripens and opens to approximately four centimetres in diameter. This phase can take several days, or it can happen very quickly. The contractions are usually irregular during this stage.

2. In the *opening phase* – also referred to as the active phase – the contractions will open the cervix up from four to ten centimetres. The contractions are usually regular during this phase.

3. The *pushing phase* starts when the cervix is completely open above the baby's head. The baby is pushed out by using the abdominal muscles, the uterine contractions and the pelvic floor.

4. The *final stage* of labour begins after the baby is born and lasts until the placenta has been pushed out.

THE BEGINNING OF LABOUR

No two births begin in exactly the same way. I know that this might be very frustrating to hear for the first-time mother who wants clear answers, but this is also what makes the whole birth process so magical. Every single childbirth brings its own unique variation and experience. The best advice I can give is to call the midwife and consult with her when you feel worried or have questions. Many women wonder how to recognize the beginning of labour. Try not to have any preconceived ideas of how it should happen. Be in the moment and take things as they come. Don't judge yourself. It's not a sign of failure if you mistake the signals and aren't as dilated as you had hoped.

Labour might start with:
- An ache similar to menstrual pains.
- The release of the mucus plug. It can look like a gel filled with blood, or it can be more like a lump of mucus. If there is plenty of blood and a persistent ache you should call a midwife and consult with her. The mucus plug is sometimes released weeks before delivery. A released mucus plug does not automatically mean you are in labour.
- The breaking of the amniotic sac. This might happen as a dramatic 'poof' with water rushing out like a waterfall, or it can be slow and dripping. The water can be clear or it can have a slight pinkish hue.
- The beginning of contractions. They can be anywhere from 15 to 90 seconds long. Commonly, they are subtle and short in the beginning. The rest periods between the contractions are usually irregular as well. The labour could, however, start off with regular contractions of 60 seconds right away.

All of these things might occur. The signals might be subtle in the beginning. It is important to remember to let the process take place in its own time. Do not get stressed or frustrated if you cannot read all the signs, or if you feel you do not understand exactly what is happening. Let the birth start in peace.

WHEN IT'S TIME TO GO

It's difficult to pinpoint the exact moment when it's time to go to the hospital or birthing centre. Many first-time mothers go too early since they do not have any previous experiences to go by. Understand that this may happen to you as well. However, the four tools can help you stay at home a little longer. Knowing when to go to the hospital can be difficult to judge, even for experienced mothers, since the body might not do what it has done during previous births. If in doubt, you should call the hospital you are assigned to, or the midwife who will come to your house if you are to deliver in your home. They will help you to interpret the signals.

One general rule is that you should go to the hospital when you have regular contractions. This means that the rushes are about 60 seconds long and keep coming every two or three minutes. For an experienced mother, it might be good to leave a little earlier, since the signs from the body can be varied.

THE FIRST PHASE

The Latent Phase
The latent phase is the first phase of childbirth. The body prepares for the coming delivery by fine-tuning all the necessary functions. This phase is like a telegram from the body telling you how you will have

to start working together soon. This phase allows you time to prepare so that you have a maximum of support and strength to last the whole labour.

During this stage of labour, the cervix opens to approximately three or four centimetres. The rushes are generally irregular and the breaks in between can be short or long. The cervix feels somewhat like a nose when you touch it with your fingers. In the early stages of labour the cervix is often tilted back, and is firm to the touch. The purpose of pain at this stage is to soften and reduce the cervix.

The first thing that happens during the contractions is that the muscles of the uterus move the edges of the cervix to the side. The cervical opening is then directed towards the front of the vagina. All of this is in preparation for the coming delivery. When the cervical opening is ready, it will start to open up to around three or four centimetres as the uterus contracts.

During the latent phase, the baby prepares by tucking its chin towards the chest and turning its body in the direction of the mother's pelvis. The baby is ready to start the journey when the cervix is completely open and wrapped around its head.

Emotions During The Latent Phase

A woman can be completely unaware of what her body is doing during this phase, or she can feel it quite strongly. The sensation of the rushes at this point can be mild and feel like an ache in the pelvic floor. This ache will later transform into a more painful sensation in the same region. But, as mentioned previously, the sensation can be quite strong even in this early stage.

Many women feel happy, excited and filled with expectation as they feel the first rushes. It is of course very exciting to be so close to meeting the baby. This is, however, a time when a lot of women wear themselves out by mentally focusing all their energy on the upcoming birth. To preserve energy, it is important not to waste it on every rush, thinking about how long it is going to take or how long the breaks are or if the labour has started or not. Think of it as a secret that only you know. This secret is slowly unravelling in your body. Every now and then you can register the rhythm of the contractions. Spend the time in between focusing on other things. Try to distract yourself as much as possible.

One couple I was assisting loved to go and look at houses that were for sale and actually spent the first part of labour viewing properties while the rushes came and went. When they returned home they relaxed in front of the television. As the labour finally got intense, the woman felt she had a lot of mental strength left. She ended up giving birth that same night.

A variety of emotions might surface during the latent phase. The woman might feel elated and happy, now that labour has finally started. She might feel confused or frustrated. Did it start for real, or not? If the pain gets severe she might feel scared. If the latent phase goes on for a long time, she might get exhausted. She might go through times when she feels distrust in her body or worries about her body's ability to handle childbirth – especially if she sees no progress in spite of the contractions. But women can also feel empowered by the ability to focus, rest and prepare, in spite of a long first phase of birth.

THE SECOND PHASE
The Opening Phase
The second phase of labour is the active opening phase. The cervix is

now three or four centimetres dilated. The contractions are more or less regular and rhythmical. Now, the rushes have the task of softly and rhythmically opening the cervix to a full ten centimetres in diameter. As the rushes move you closer and closer to the goal they intensify and the feeling of pressure increases.

A pushing sensation can sometimes occur in the opening phase before the woman is fully dilated. If this happens it can be necessary to help the body to stop actively pushing by holding back the sensation rather than following it through. This can be done by lying down with the bottom up in the air so that the pressure lessens and the urge to push subsides.

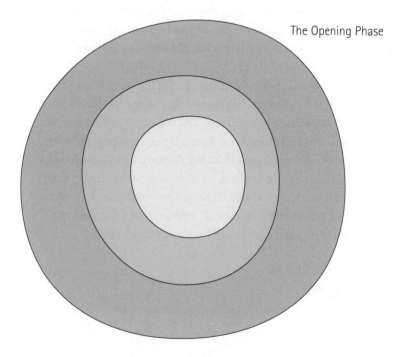

The Opening Phase

It can be difficult to comprehend what is happening and why it has to hurt. Visualization can help you to understand how the contractions work to open up the cervix. I suggest using the image of a rubber band, softly widening in harmony with the rushes. Visualize how it stretches and elongates to help the baby through. This will help you understand the purpose of the sensation. What you are experiencing is not in any way harmful. At the end of the opening phase, the cervix is dilated to ten centimetres and is placed right above the baby's head.

The baby is now starting its labourious journey out into the world. The baby slowly moves down the birth canal one contraction at a time, adapting to the shape of the pelvis and vagina by twisting and turning the body. The baby rotates and works to assist you in your effort.

The baby will pass a place in the pelvis called the ischial spine. This is the narrowest part of the pelvis. In some women this causes nausea. As the baby moves deeper and further down the birth canal towards the opening of the vagina and pushes onto the pelvic floor, the contractions will shift and the urge to bear down and push gets more intense.

Emotions During The Opening Phase

Some women experience the opening phase as chaotic and hard to comprehend. The problem is that this phase is not always clear and distinct. It is not possible to see or feel what the uterus and cervix are doing. A woman might feel a sensation of pain and it might be hard to know what to do about it, and what the purpose is. Some women find this phase very easy to deal with as there is no requirement to do anything. The woman simply has to let go, whereas the pushing phase that follows requires effort.

The most important thing in the opening phase is experiencing the immediate *now*. It is about the contraction you are sensing right *now*, or the break you are in right *now*. If you start pondering the number of contractions you might have left, or how long it is going to take, you will have to deal with more than one contraction. You are carrying them all at the same time. Notions of time only make the process unmanageable. It is important that all the people around help to keep the focus on what is behind you, not in front of you. The thought of being in pain for another two hours might be unbearable. If you instead shift your perspective and deal with the present you will be able to handle a lot more than you could imagine. Be mindful and remind yourself to collect your thoughts throughout the process of giving birth.

During the opening phase the woman might still feel confused and wonder if the labour has started or not. She might, however, feel a sense of empowerment from being able to handle the force of the contractions. First-time mothers who have no reference points usually have the notion that the labour has progressed further along than it actually has.

When the delivery accelerates the woman might temporarily react with despair. She will have to adjust to the increased force. If she allows time to settle into this new phase, she will regain confidence and feel secure again. If the birth up until this point has been more drawn out than expected, it might feel like a heavy burden to think about how difficult the process can be and how much still lies ahead. It is common to swing between positive and negative emotions.

THE THIRD PHASE
The Pushing Phase
The third and last phase of labour is the pushing phase. This phase starts

when the baby has finished the journey down the birth canal and has its head right by the pelvic floor. There can be an overwhelming urge to bear down. Many women feel as though they are going to have a bowel movement, or like there is a heavy pressure towards their bottom. However, some women have more diffused sensations that are harder to define. There are women who feel overtaken by the rushes at this stage and all they can to do is to give in and push. It can sometimes be a less pronounced force, especially if the woman has received an epidural.

The uterus, the pelvic floor and the abdominal muscles all participate in the pushing phase. The muscle threads making up the pelvic floor are able to contract and relax simultaneously. The ability to contract and relax makes them strong, yet elastic.

When the baby's head has reached the vagina, the only thing left is the passage through the opening. The contractions press the baby's head towards the opening, which increasingly gets wider as the contractions continue. It is very common for the baby's head to retract back after a contraction. This allows the mother and baby to have a chance to recover and for the tissue to get more elastic. Finally the baby's head has expanded the vagina to a point where the head does not retract after a rush. This is a sign that the actual birth is very close.

Once the head has stretched the opening to a point where it is wide enough, the child's whole head will come through. Sometimes the body follows during the same contraction. Other times the head will emerge during one contraction and the body during the next.

Emotions During The Pushing Phase

The pushing phase is often more tangible than the opening phase. The pain has shifted and the rushes work more clearly to move the baby out.

This part of the labour can be a relief since the woman can actually feel what is happening, though it can also be frightening since the pressure is so enormous. The pushing phase requires her to take an active part and the challenge is to follow along. The pressure on the pelvic floor can give you the sensation that you need to go to the toilet. This might lead to you squeezing your muscles and working against your body. Just because you feel like you need to defecate it doesn't mean you will, and if you do, the staff will take care of it in a discreet way. Try to affirm the sensation and do not hold back.

This is also the stage when many women think of the impossibility of something that big coming out of something that narrow. Just because you feel a certain way, it does not mean that it is true. The vagina is made up of pleated mucus membrane. It is constructed to be able to widen and let the baby through, and then pull back to a normal size.

Envision how it wraps tightly around the baby. The vagina has the ability to stretch and become surprisingly large. Ina May Gaskin, a famous American midwife, makes a funny comparison in her book *Ina May's Guide to Childbirth*. She questions why we never ask how a penis can go from small to big and small again without permanent damage. A woman's sexual organs have the same ability to increase in size and then retract.

There are many different opinions on the best way to avoid tearing while pushing the baby out. These issues are important, but I think the most important thing is for the woman to get help in handling her fears. Fear will affect the elasticity of the muscles and tissues in a negative way. A pelvic floor resisting and tightening will not let a baby through. If the mother has a sense of trust and the atmosphere around her is supportive and calm, the blood circulation to the muscles and tissues will increase and the baby will be able to pass through.

Various emotions will come and go during the pushing phase. You might be filled with energy since you will soon be meeting the baby. You might get scared since the pressure can be overwhelming. Or it may feel wonderful that something is finally happening. The impulse to bear down may overcome you and your body. You might find yourself incapable of holding back even when trying your hardest. You might get the feeling that you will not be able to go through with it even though your body is working at top capacity. Right afterwards you might be in a state of shock. You will need time to come back down to earth and to get to know your newborn baby.

FEAR OF LACERATIONS

It comes as no surprise that women fear lacerations. The thought of one's genitals rupturing is terrifying. However, this is a misleading description, and it is almost as if we have taught ourselves to think in a negative and terrifying way. The pelvic floor is designed to be able to adjust itself to accommodate the baby's journey. This accommodation sometimes includes a natural laceration. The shape of the vagina and the tissues surrounding it are made to be able to tear a little to make the passing of the baby smoother. They are also designed to heal quickly. It is not a big deal. Women often do not even notice a laceration occurring during birth. The genitals might feel sore after a vaginal birth, whether you had a laceration or not. We need to erase the old negative way of looking at this, and actively embrace a new way of seeing it as something normal.

A woman needs support and help during the pushing phase so that she does not get caught up in fear and stress, which could exacerbate the problem and cause more extensive tears. Let the pushing take its time. Fear will tighten the muscles, causing the birth process to halt until you are in a safe place. To reduce these emotions you need to be in a calm, safe and unforced environment. Listen to the instructions of the midwife and let her know you want to take your time.

Many women fear the pushing phase. It is hard to understand how something so big can come out of something so small. The pushing phase is the most intense part of the delivery and is therefore obviously the scariest. This fear is also based on ignorance. As I mentioned before, the vagina is made up of pleated mucus membrane that has the ability to expand in size. The vagina can get really big if you are relaxed and safe, and then go back to its normal size again. Use the information to shift your inner picture and expand your limitations. You do not have to believe this part to be easy. What you can do is use the tools to give the body the support it needs, and to prevent your energy being used up by working against the process.

exercise

Preparing for a confident birth:
Reduce the fear of lacerations

- Shift your perspective and look at a small laceration as a natural part of giving birth.
- Prevent larger tears by allowing yourself to take time, by not getting scared and by making sure you are safe.
- Understand how you are built. The body is made to be able to handle all parts of childbirth. Build faith around this.

AFTER DELIVERY

After the child is born there is a break in the contractions before it's time for the placenta to be delivered. It can take anything from a few minutes up to an hour. When the placenta has detached from the uterus wall, the uterus will contract to push the placenta out. This feels like a contraction, but the placenta is soft and will easily pass through the opening of the vagina. When this is done, the midwife can massage the mother's stomach to help the uterus shrink back. She will also look to see if there are any ruptures or tears that need to be repaired.

LENGTH OF THE DELIVERY

Each delivery consists of all these phases, but each labour varies greatly in length and intensity. Some women never feel the latent phase, and start off their labour in the opening phase. Other women have a prolonged latent phase. There are cases when the cervix opens to ten centimetres very quickly, only to come to a halt while the body takes a break and recharges before the pushing contractions start. The opening phase might be very long and drawn out only to be followed by a short pushing phase.

Even though it might be very difficult for us to acknowledge that there are areas of our lives that cannot be controlled, we have to accept that we have no control over the process of childbirth. It is a dimension of life that is not bound by laws of time and space, but guided by different principles. As a general rule a first-time mother has a longer delivery, and the phases are a little more drawn out, though this is not always true. The second child usually comes quicker. But as always, there are exceptions and you should keep your mind open to whatever happens.

A MOTHER IS BORN

When the delivery is over, your new life as a mother begins. It takes time to make this adjustment, both physically and mentally, and various emotions and feelings will come and go. Some women feel elated. For other women it takes a while to discover their mothering and nurturing instincts.

Women are often very sensitive and emotional after giving birth. This is because the mother needs to be emotionally available to be able to bond with her new baby. This emotional openness makes her vulnerable. Therefore you are not meant to meet a lot of people, or to be too active. If you wait a few days, you will have had a chance to bond with the baby and you will be a little stronger and more resilient.

The body can be sore after the delivery and you need a lot of peace and quiet. Everything can feel new, but have faith in your ability to take care of the baby and learn how to breastfeed.

There is nothing wrong, even if you don't know everything from the beginning. Overcoming the difficulties and solving problems will build up your confidence as a parent. You are the mother of this baby and you have all the capacity you need to take care of him or her, even if you do not know all the details.

Do not hesitate to ask for advice or support when you need it. It does not mean you are failing. A positive outlook does not mean you never ask for help, but rather that you assume you are capable of handling what comes, even if it is not perfect all the time.

Gabriella's birth story

April 13th
00.00 on the hour:
At the hospital. Relax. I am here now. I like the room. The warm, friendly staff greet me. It only takes midwife Lina five minutes to 'get me'. What a relief! A midwife in training is right next to Lina. I say it's okay if she wants to stay. I am four centimetres dilated now. I change clothes, put on the gown, walk with the walker in the corridor. I stop and breathe into every rush, sinking into it. It is not hard. We walk around, laughing and talking in between contractions. After half an hour I want to retreat to the room and not see people. I just want to be cocooned in the comfort of the delivery room. Richard quietly takes on the role of the protector, coach and support.

We decided beforehand that I would use my hands to gesture when I could feel a contraction. When I raise my hand everything has to go quiet and calm. Juice with a straw, water, pillows; he gets me whatever I need and keeps close to me. I cannot communicate with words. I need to sink deeply into myself. He understands. I feel how he is right there with me – not feeling excluded. It is priceless to know that I do not have to explain myself, or complicate things by saying 'please, could you help my by...' because there is no way I could find the time between contractions.

I feel the love and support from his hands when he massages my shoulders and firmly brings his hands down along my body. It calms me, brings me closer to the earth, gets the oxytocin flowing in me. Staying with the contractions. Managing them all on my own. I dare to sink into each rush, dive into myself and momentarily lose myself. I say quietly to myself 'Yes, baby, down, out, out, out and down. I love you and you are welcome to this world' during each contraction. Suddenly the contractions intensify – I can feel a barrier now. It is a barrier of fear, a deep fear from the bottom of my soul. It is mine and I have to face it. I see it. It has a shape to it. Like a see-through floor, tinted red. I know I have to go through it to see the ground, but I seem to bounce back without the ability to go through it. A moment of panic – I cannot go down, I dare not to sink all the way. I know the only way to get this baby out is to dive even deeper into myself, to give in to the pain. I need the support of our doula – I trust her to guide me through the barrier of fear.

02.00

My doula arrives at 02.00. She is all calm, strength and experience. I trust her fully. The first thing she does after saying hello is to turn the radio off. 'Aha', I think to myself, 'I was trying to escape through the music!' I have to give this 100% if it is to work. The room is silent now. My confidence returns and I feel safe as she touches me, caressing my hands and body. Softly, calmly she guides me down into myself. She is there during each contraction. I can talk and think between the contractions now. I observe myself from the outside. The redness of the fear evaporates when she assists me during the contractions. I now see light as I close my eyes. The light is the guiding light. The pain is even more intense now, but I am completely calm inside. I am able to let go more and more. The atmosphere in the room is of great importance – it has to be absolutely quiet during the contractions for me to be able to go deep inside and disappear. Something feels wrong – the trainee midwife is giving off too much energy. She is all revved up and her energy is not in sync with the grounded, calming mood I need to surround myself with. I feel bad, but I have to express my feelings. I ask Lina the midwife if she can tell her student to move back.

Lina understands completely and I let go of that thought. I am once again calm and peaceful.

03.00
Six centimetres dilated now. I discover that the more I am able to let my feelings, my body and my mind go the easier it gets. I have the courage to find a position where I tilt my head back with my chin up towards the ceiling, as if I was surrendering. Arms hanging loose, palms up, almost like I am meditating. This makes it easier for me to breathe through the contractions. Previously I was leaning forward when the rush came – like I was trying to protect myself or hide. Instead I give in. Nothing else exists. Richard massages my back firmly during the contractions. It feels as if the baby is ready to come out through my spine.

I take a very hot bath. Running water – the sound helps me to let go of everything around me. Richard is positioned behind me. He has cold towels – ready to cool my forehead and chest between the rushes. My doula is right next to me. She is holding my hand through the pain. Guiding me. The world is fading more and more.

I am completely calm and secure. I get all the help and undivided focus I need to be able to fold into myself. Every ounce of panic that surfaces is swiftly overcome by the soft voice of my doula. During each rush she reminds me to relax with her mantra: 'Relax your eyebrows, soften your jaw, loosen your chin, relax your shoulders.' Richard starts chanting 'Yeeeeesss'. In the midst of this it hits me – how I feel like I am in a monastery in Tibet. The thought makes me smile. This deep, repeating chant helps me to stay grounded. I sing along with him, seeking the depth of his tone.

The pain is shifting. It wants to move out and down. I need to stand up. I sit on the toilet for a few minutes. Welcoming the rushes with my breath. It is four a.m. It is starting to bear down. I recognize the sensation. The pushing contractions are about to start soon. I move to the bed. I lean forward on a pillow by my belly. NOW I am completely overtaken by the excruciating force. I feel like I am about to explode. It does not end, I cannot breathe. I just have time to think 'Help me. I cannot take this any longer. I want laughing gas'. My doula is repeating 'Yeeess, Yeeeess'. Now all I can do is push, push, pushing out. I am not using the laughing gas. There is no time. Suddenly – that burning, piercing pain. The head is fixed. I am holding on to Richard and my doula for all I am worth. The pressure is immense. The force is ripping me apart. Her words ring in my ears: 'You can do this, everything is alright, he is going to be here soon, push him out'. She repeats this over and over again. Then 'SPLASH!' His whole body is emerging in one push. A scream. Warmth is rushing from me. No more pain. I can breathe. I listen for him. Listen to everybody's reactions. Is he healthy? Does he have all his parts? He has a short umbilical cord, so they cut it. I get help to turn around. Our miracle is resting on my chest. So beautiful! So you were the one inside of me waiting to come and see me? My beloved son, welcome to this world!

13 minutes of pushing. It felt like an eternity. Our little prince was born at 04.18 a.m.

2

The four tools

You will now get to familiarize yourself with the four tools –
breathing, **relaxation**, **sound**, and the **power of the mind**.
Imagine the tools as steps on a staircase that you slowly walk
down during labour. When the rushes come, you start with the
breathing. During the first stage of labour you might only work
with the breathing. As the contractions get more intense, you take
the breathing with you down to the next step, relaxation. When
you have walked down all the steps, the tools will melt together
and stay with you. Your breathing is calm and you are relaxed. For
the last part of the birth, and through your pushes, you use your
voice and the power of your mind. These four tools will lead you
down towards your goal, welcoming the baby into the world.

Introducing the four tools

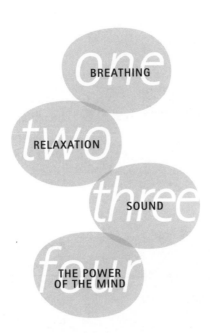

BREATHING

RELAXATION

SOUND

**THE POWER
OF THE MIND**

These tools are only to be used during the contractions. Use the space in between rushes for resting and simply being in the moment. The tools are not dependent on, or tied together with specific phases of labour. You can choose to use them whenever you like when facing a contraction. You might also want to use only one of them during labour. They all work very well on their own.

You might get the impression that these tools are simple and obvious when you practise using them during your pregnancy. But what might seem simple and obvious now, can be difficult and easy to forget if you get scared and overcome by fear. Do not underestimate the importance of practice.

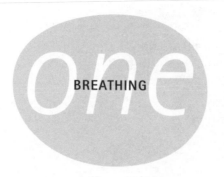

BREATHING

Your **BREATHING** is directly connected to your feelings. By breathing calmly you will get a positive feeling, which reduces stress and fear.

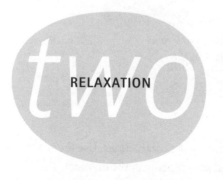

RELAXATION

RELAXATION is the opposite of stress and will help you to stay calm through your contractions. This will reduce tension and prevent you from working against yourself during labour.

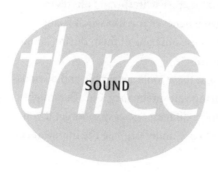

SOUND

The **SOUND** of your voice can be of great help in preventing fear and stress. A deep voice will also engage your abdominal muscles, which in turn will assist you during the pushing phase.

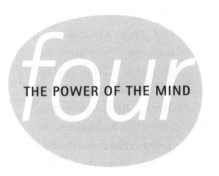

THE POWER OF THE MIND

The **POWER OF THE MIND** can help you to access your inner resources of optimism, trust and faith. These resources will be there for you during labour, and when you are facing pain.

Some tools might come easily to you, and others might feel more alien. Do not be afraid of the ones that feel strange or unfamiliar. Sometimes what works best during labour might be something you thought you wouldn't use at all. Often it is hard to intellectualize what makes the tools work; you simply know that they do.

CREATING A FEELING OF SECURITY

Security is the opposite of fear. The four tools create a feeling of security to break the automatic chain of response connected to fear. You feel safe and secure when you know that what is happening to you is not damaging or harmful. The body's reward system kicks in, blood circulation increases, the reproductive organs get more energy and you feel happier. The breathing becomes softer and quieter, the muscles relax, the voice deepens and the mind calms down. To be able to stimulate relaxation and security, and thereby lessen the negative emotions which make the birthing process harder, I try to lead the woman through the body's own natural manifestations of security and confidence: gentle breathing, relaxed muscles, a deep voice and positive thoughts. As you can see, they are using the natural connection between body and emotion. All the emotions have their own way of manifesting themselves in the body. Through this connection you can transport your body to a state of calmness, which will in turn affect your feelings. You already have all of these connections – all you have to do is show the way.

To illustrate this I would like you to imagine getting a contraction. When you start sensing the contraction you might automatically tense up. By doing this you risk ending up in a negative cycle. Try to relax as soon as you feel the contraction. This might be the opposite of your first impulse. If, in spite of feeling the force of the contraction, you are able to relax your jaw, relax your shoulders, breathe deeper and more gently, the sensation of fear will not arise. You are guiding your feelings away from fear towards safety and confidence. When using the reversed response to fear, it gets harder for the body to descend into emotions of fear and stress.

This is how easily the anti-stress model works; it is easy but sometimes it is also quite difficult. It takes both knowledge and practice to master the technique, and you need to learn how to be brave and relax while in what can sometimes be a difficult and frightening situation. However, when you finally take the steps needed and feel the difference, you will not want to go back.

Pain can trigger an automatic chain reaction.
It might look like the following:

1. Pain.
2. Reaction: Tension, saying no, wanting to escape.
3. End result: Cramping and locking up.

You can break this chain reaction by using the four tools. This will stimulate positive feelings. It looks like this:

1. Pain.
2. Reaction: Relaxing, saying Yes! Staying in the moment.
3. Result: The confidence to give birth.

PHYSICAL EXPRESSIONS OF
FEAR AND CONFIDENCE

When I started working with labouring women, I discovered how many times they were unaware of the negative stress pattern they were caught up in. Instead I learned to recognise it by studying their body language. As time went on I developed a sensibility towards this, and the body became my most important instrument in helping these women.

Every emotion has its very own unique physical expression. To be able to use the four tools you need to understand how fear manifests itself in the body. In this way you can quickly break the cycle.

However, it is not enough to understand the negative reactions. You also have to be aware of the positive reaction patterns, as this is what the tools are based upon. These bodily expressions are the opposite of stress. Opposite is a list of the most common physical signals of fear and stress, and calmness and confidence.

RECEIVING THE CONTRACTIONS

The tools presented in this book will help you to activate the body's own pain inhibitors. This system is accessible to help you, and it kicks in when you feel confident and safe. However, if your focus is only to muffle the pain you're feeling, these techniques could have the opposite effect and instead work against the whole birthing process. You should try to focus on working with and facing up to the pain. The pain will get more and more intense during labour, regardless of what pain medication you use. It's supposed to work this way. The pain is caused by the uterus working towards giving birth to the baby.

It might not always feel like a positive thing, but the force is always positive in the end. It is what helps a woman to welcome her baby. If

Fear and stress

Fear and stress are manifested in one or a combination of the following ways.

During contractions:
- Loud and forced breathing
- Tense shoulders, clenched jaw, tight hands
- Shifting gaze, body in movement
- Difficulty in being still
- Tendency to push up with the hands and lifting the body upwards from the bedding
- Standing on tiptoes
- A high-pitched and strained voice

Between contractions:
- Difficulty relaxing
- Difficulty sleeping and resting, sometimes for several days
- Negative emotions and resignation for an extended time

Calmness and confidence

These can be one or a combination of the following.

During contractions:
- Calm and quiet breathing
- Heavy and relaxed body
- Closed or focused eyes
- Willingness not to control or fight the contractions, and just go with the flow.
- Deep and calm voice

Between contractions:
- Relaxed and centred between rushes
- Ability to sleep and rest when tired
- Emotions that come and go naturally

you are trying to slow down or curb this force, you end up working against your body. Instead of making you feel stronger, it will make you lose faith in your own ability. To avoid this, your preparation needs to include strategies to handle the pain, not just to lessen it. In order to face up to pain it's necessary to welcome it and allow it to come closer. Imagine a wave washing over your body. It rushes in, takes over, and then subsides.

With the help of these tools you will be able to flow along with the course of events in peace with your body. You can't control or change what happens, but the tools will help you to welcome the pain and the force of the contractions. Regardless of the choice of pain medication, you will probably experience some pain. The sensation gets stronger and more powerful the closer you get to the goal – the birth of the baby. But what is threatening is not pain itself. It's the fear.

I was present at a birth where the woman was afraid to move around. The pain got stronger every time she shifted position. She took a bath and became more and more motionless. I encouraged her to move around, even though it was more painful for her. We made up a plan to help her to deal with the contractions. Instead of tensing up, she would flow along with the contractions and whatever movements she could detect.

When the contractions came, I encouraged her to welcome them. I kept repeating that everything was as it should be, and that her body was helping her reach the end result. She stepped out of the bath, and as soon as she felt the contractions she put her head back, made a deep sound and swayed her hips. It worked! She felt powerful and her self-confidence grew since she knew she had the ability to face the force of the contractions.

HANDLING THE CONTRACTIONS WITH THE TOOLS

You do not have to teach your body to give birth by reading or working out. All you have to do to bring out this inherent wisdom is to focus on two things: the contractions and the tools.

At the end of the day we will never know how the delivery is going to develop; how it will start or end. We can always guess, but you cannot control or foresee it. However, we do know that there are going to be contractions. It is difficult to predict if they will be effective, what phase they are in and how they will feel. But we do know that there will be contractions from the start until the end of labour. So, to help your body and to create a feeling of positive control, you and your partner can focus on handling one contraction at a time by using the four simple tools.

These tools emanate from basic physiological principles leading the body away from stress and fear and towards its fantastic ability to give birth.

So, my beautiful friend, what if it could be easy to give birth? Not easy as in no challenges, or void of pain, or everything working as planned. No, easy in a way where you can use the tools to take away resistance so that you use all your strength to work with your amazing body, rather than against it.

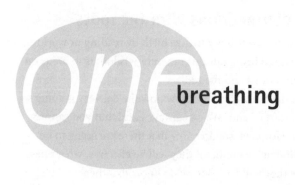

breathing

I have been engaged as a doula for Moa and Axel. When I arrive at their apartment I discover that Moa hasn't slept for 24 hours. She tells me that she is extremely tired and exhausted. She keeps repeating this over and over and I can sense her desperation. I watch her as she is having a contraction. She is sitting down on a chair with another chair facing her. As the rushes gets stronger, her breathing can be heard throughout the whole room. I can see how her breathing pattern creates fear in her body. The typical signs are there: her body is restless, her toes are trying to grasp the floor, she is frowning, her shoulders are high up and there is a general sense of tightness throughout her whole body. I crawl right up to her, very close. I lean my forehead against hers and I whisper that her breathing needs to be adjusted. I talk to her softly, using a deep voice through her next contraction. I tell her that her breathing is too loud and that she needs to breathe softly and calmly. I explain that I'll assist her in breathing soundlessly. I stay right there with her and as soon as I hear her breathing becoming forced, I remind her to breathe softly and calmly. Slowly her breathing gets quieter and becomes inaudible. She is breathing more and more softly and she lets each exhalation pour out from her body without a sound. The whole time we work together to make her breathing calmer and more passive so that her body can relax. Before long she can feel the results. The contractions grow gentler and she is less scared. She is fascinated and surprised at the difference in the sensation. I keep guiding her and after a while she is relaxed enough to fall asleep. She is able to rest for a few hours and when she wakes up labour has finally kicked in. Her contractions are powerful and when we get to the hospital she is six centimetres dilated.

As we have seen, breathing is closely connected to a woman's feelings. All the emotions are manifested in your breathing. You sigh when satisfied, hold your breath if scared, and start hyperventilating if you have to escape. The most noticeable signs of fear during labour often get expressed through the breathing patterns. It is common to hold the breath during the contractions. Many women also believe intense, audible breathing is soothing. They are under the impression that they need to oxygenate the blood for the baby as much as possible. The balance between oxygen and carbon dioxide is sensitive and might get disturbed by forceful breathing. The pain and stress get more intense from all the breathing and this in turn creates agony, which in turn creates hyperventilation and anxiety. A bad cycle is created.

You need to find a natural way of breathing to be able to break this negative cycle. I always start with the breathing when helping a woman in stress. It is the most effective tool when dealing with fear.

NATURAL BREATHING

The most important elements of natural breathing are that it should be soft, soundless and without tension. The breathing is calm and mild when you feel relaxed and safe. This calm breathing goes deep into the abdomen, and it makes you relaxed and secure. During inhalation you use the muscles to fill the lungs. This is the active part of breathing. The exhalation is completely passive. The air streams and flows out without you having to use any muscle power. While exhaling, the muscles relax, and the shoulders drop.

By breathing in a calm and relaxed way during labour, the body will find its organic breathing pattern, which will keep stress reactions at bay. You do not need to put much effort into this, since organic breathing comes naturally and automatically

SOUNDLESS BREATHING

In reality, the way in which you breathe does not matter all that much while you are in labour, as long as the breathing is calm and soundless. If you are breathing in this way the body will take over and create its own rhythm. It does not matter whether you inhale through your mouth or your nose. In my opinion, the more you think of how to breathe, the more difficult it gets. Your body will find what works best for you according to how the baby is positioned and how deep or shallow you need to breathe.

A woman once told me she thought it was hard to breathe soundlessly during her contractions. Her instinct was to breathe forcefully and strongly. This raises an important point which is that the four tools can be used to manipulate your instinctive response. Fear is connected to this response and causes the breathing to become faster in an effort to oxygenate the muscles in preparation for flight. The uterus does not need the same amount of oxygen as the whole muscle system. The increased breathing only serves to build tension and fear. By breathing softly and soundlessly you can counteract this reaction. This will make it harder to tip over into stressed and forced breathing and ultimately lose control.

It is not difficult to keep your breathing calm and soundless. The instructions in the exercises will help you to learn how to listen to your breathing. Your breath should not be heard in the room. Let the feeling remind you of a quiet wind, blowing through your system. Let the breath flow free. *The most important thing is to listen. If you think you can hear your breath in the room, try to make your breathing as quiet and soft as possible.*

Practising breathing during pregnancy

If you work consciously with the breathing cycle it can make the breathing feel strained and jagged. Do not try to change things, just try to explore and observe. Focus on relaxing and feeling comfortable.

STEP 1. If you listen to your breathing while reading you can get a sense of how it sounds when you are free from fear. Put the book away and observe how you are breathing. How does it sound? Where in your body can you feel your breath? What happens during the exhalation? What happens to your shoulders and your body? What goes on while you inhale? Repeat a few times.

▼

STEP 2. Try breathing loudly and with force, so that you can hear your inhalations and exhalations vibrating in the room. Exaggerate a few times. Did it change your feelings? How did your body feel? How long can you keep going before you start to feel dizzy? What is the biggest difference in comparison to the soundless breathing?

STEP 3. Go back to the soundless, calm and soft breathing. Let your exhalations be soft, gradual and pleasant. Use the breathing in a way that feels good. Repeat a few times. How does this feel? Emotionally? Physically?

Ask your support person to listen so that he or she can hear the difference.

Techniques during contractions

These techniques should be used for the entire length of the contraction.

1. Relax the lips and the jaw. This is so as not to tighten the mouth.
2. Keep the inhalations soft and inaudible. The purpose of this is to keep the shoulders down.
3. Breathe out slowly and softly. Exhalations are naturally longer than inhalations. Let them be as slow and smooth as possible. Try to put the brakes on a little to slow them down. The body sinks and relaxes downwards while breathing out.

If you find it difficult to breathe slowly, you might want to increase the speed of the breathing for a while, but remember to keep the inhalations and exhalations soft and soundless. Do it your own way if you have difficulty following the instructions, but keep the basic principles in mind – soft and soundless. Go back to your normal, natural breathing when the contraction eases off. Let your breath flow free, the way it needs to.

OTHER BREATHING TECHNIQUES

You can apply the method of breathing softly and soundlessly to yoga breathing, Lamaze, or any other breathing technique you choose to use.

The French obstetrician Fernand Lamaze invented the prophylaxis breathing technique, which is a commonly used method. By practising specific breathing patterns, the woman can manipulate the body's conditioned responses. Lamaze assigned several particular ways of breathing to correspond with the three stages of labour. These breathing patterns are intended to make pain management easier. Lamaze's techniques sometimes go by the name *profylax*, a Swedish word meaning prevention or preparation, though it is used in a variety of contexts. The common goal for all the different breathing techniques is to maintain the balance between oxygen and carbon dioxide, which helps you to relax. I have chosen to use a simpler breathing technique, which works in a similar way to Lamaze. Since it doesn't give you specific advice on *how* to breathe you can use my suggestions for calm and soundless breathing with any technique you choose to follow.

CONCLUDING THE CONTRACTION WITH A SIGH

The most important part of breathing is the sigh. You sigh with satisfaction and relief because it feels good! When relaxed and secure you sigh several times an hour without even noticing. When you sigh your shoulders drop, and your neck and face relax and become soft. This does not occur when you are stressed or scared and it leaves your muscles tense. In today's hectic society we often feel aches and pains in our body. This is what happens when the natural way of relaxing is being blocked off.

Sighing is a natural way of relaxing during labour. After the contraction subsides it can be hard to get rid of the built-up tension. You unconsciously keep tensing up, and resting becomes impossible. By sighing after each contraction you can neutralize the tension and relax the body. By doing this you also create a downward movement and this automatically makes the body more relaxed.

Practising before the birth

- Put the book away and explore what happens as you sigh.
- Try slowly filling your lungs.
- Sigh with or without sound.
- Try to make sounds with your mouth closed and then with your mouth open.
- Try 'aaaaah' or 'mmmmm' for example.

When you sigh, both before and afterwards, note what happens to the shoulders, the face, and the arms. Can you exaggerate the movement? Try a couple of times.

Practise after each contraction

- Finish each contraction by filling the lungs and then exhaling with a deep sigh. Repeat one or two times.
- The sigh can be soundless, or you can make a 'haaaaa' sound.
- Do not be afraid to exaggerate!
- Be aware of relaxing your shoulders and becoming heavy when you exhale.

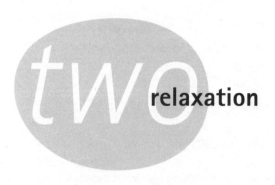

relaxation

I work at the maternity ward as an assistant nurse. Today, my workday starts with Lena and Mats. Lena has been labouring for over 24 hours and she has not slept at all during that time. She is inhaling laughing gas when I enter the room. She gets up on tiptoes during the contractions and her whole body is pulling upwards. She keeps repeating how tired she is. After a while I feel like we have a connection. I suggest that she does things a little differently this time so that she can also get some rest. I tell her she has to let go of the laughing gas for a short while, but that she can come right back to it if she doesn't like what we're doing. It is a little frightening to leave the laughing gas at first, but she is very tired and ready to try almost anything. I shut the blinds and turn off the light. I place her half seated on the bed, with a pillow behind her neck. Then we start. As the contraction comes I help her to slowly release and get heavy, to melt into the bedding. With every breath I talk to her about getting heavy, being brave and relaxing her shoulders and jaw. I keep encouraging her to be in the moment, to be heavy and relaxed as the contraction approaches. I adjust her breathing, making it soft and soundless. We breathe together

and I repeat 'heavy... heavy... heavy. Let your body go, and feel yourself
getting heavy... heavy... heavy'.

It only takes a few minutes until we feel the calm, silent magic in the
room. She is completely still and absolutely beautiful. I know her body still
feels the pain, but the pain has changed shape. She is now capable of being
still, letting the forces inside her work. No movement or struggle can be
seen on the surface. Since her contractions can't be seen, her husband fears
they have subsided. I whisper that they are as strong as ever, but that she
is now able to accept them. He is amazed and also impressed by her ability
to handle the contractions. Lena gives me a wonderful explanation of how
she experienced the difference.

'It is fantastic! It feels like the contractions are blowing through me now.
Earlier it was as if they severed my insides, but now it is more like a soft
wind. The pain is still there, but it is softer.'

I smile. The contractions are still there. But they are not as acute and
grinding as before. Soon she'll be able to rest, even fall asleep in between
rushes.

The foundation of all relaxation is learning to counteract stress by
experiencing the weight of the body. The feeling of heaviness will help
you to sink into the body and flow along deep down into the waves of
the contractions. It is the weight of the body that will help you to stay
in the moment and prevent you from fleeing. It is much harder to flee
when you weigh a ton than if you are on tiptoes ready to run. By feeling
the weight you will get a sensation of melting into the contraction and
staying relaxed.

The goal of the tools is to help the body to take full advantage of the
contractions. When you are scared you block the body. Fear makes

you stand on tiptoes, pull the shoulders up and talk with a shrill voice. The common denominator of the tools is that they work in the same direction as the contractions. Birth conforms to the law of gravity and moves in a downward direction. The baby moves down the birth canal, and the uterus works to help the baby on its journey.

ACTIVELY PASSIVE

You need to allow yourself to be passive and heavy during the contractions. This will help you to go along with the downward movement of the birth. In order to find the courage to become heavy and passive, you need to work actively. It might sound contradictory to be passive and active at the same time. However, using the tools is an active way of staying passive. The contractions aim downwards to help the baby out of the uterus. The four tools will help you to reinforce this movement rather than working against it.

To visualize the contraction, you should think of it as a valley, instead of as a peak, which is how contractions are normally described. It is much more strenuous to climb to the top of a peak of a mountain then it is to slide passively to the bottom of a valley. By creating a mental image of sliding softly to the bottom of the contraction, you will make it easier to flow along.

DIVING TECHNIQUE

The Swedish midwife Cayenne Ekjordh has created a technique called the 'diving technique'. She had been working as a midwife for many years when one day while on holiday she found herself caught up in a big wave in the Atlantic Ocean. She struggled hard, but soon realised that it was all in vain. In the middle of the wave she realized she had to let go and let the wave take her towards the shore. It worked. She was dazed and out of breath, but she had survived.

It took a few years before she came to the realization that this must be the way to handle the waves of the contractions. If the labouring woman lets go and gets heavy, the wave will take her to shore. From this experience she created the 'diving technique'. The diving technique helps the woman to dive into her body and the experience without fighting it. I was inspired by the diving technique when I created the first two tools.

MUSCLE TENSION

As I mentioned earlier, the body reacts to fear by a chain of automatic responses. The shoulders come up towards the ears, you make fists with your hands and your jaw gets tight. Tension also shows in the face, as a wrinkle between the eyebrows and as a tightening in the lips and around your mouth. This is how we are used to seeing birthing women on the screen. However, this is a picture of a woman in fear, and not of a woman giving birth!

The trapezius muscle – the muscle that extends over the neck, shoulders and part of the back – is very sensitive to fear. This muscle is closely tied to our emotions, in much the same way as the other muscles in the face. These muscles react to feelings of fear, flight and defence. When you are exposed to something you perceive as threatening, your emotions are activated, which automatically affects the muscles. You can break this automatic chain of response by actively working to relax the shoulders, face, brows and the entire body during the contraction. By being heavy and relaxed, you eliminate the flight response.

To give a clear picture of what I mean by being heavy and passive, imagine the sensation of sinking into water. You get heavier and heavier with each breath. Evoke a feeling of passiveness and weight in your body in different physical positions: standing up, sitting and lying down.

During the contraction you sink deep. You do not have to fall like a rock, just get the general feeling of going downwards. Lean your head against someone or something, let your arms and shoulders sink, and relax your face. Keep a space between your feet and rhythmically bend your knees so that the movement is down towards the ground. Use your exhalations to relax even more. Be mindful of your shoulders, since they can easily get tense.

exercise

Exercises during pregnancy

Lie down or lean back. Tighten and then relax different muscles. You will get to feel the difference between a tense and a relaxed muscle.

STEP 1. Tense and then relax two or three times:
1. Forehead/eyes
2. Jaw/mouth
3. Neck/shoulders
4. Arms/hands
5. Thighs/gluteal muscles (the muscles in your bottom)
6. Feet

STEP 2
1. Tense the entire body. How does it feel? What emotions come to the surface?
2. Use your exhalations to reinforce the downward movement. Start off by tensing the whole body. As you breathe out, let go of your

▼

jaw, head and shoulders. Let your arms and hands fall down and
let your whole body relax.
3. Repeat a couple of times and feel how all the stress melts away.
How does it feel? What emotion does it produce?

MUSCLES OF THE PELVIC FLOOR

There are many muscles in the pelvic floor that might be tense during
labour without the labouring women being conscious of it. If they
become too tense they can make delivery more difficult, or even
impossible. When the pelvic floor is tense, the face, jaw and mouth
are tense as well. All of the circular sphincter muscles in the body are
connected. You can use this connection to help relax the pelvic floor
during the contractions.

exercise

PELVIC FLOOR EXERCISES

Exercise during pregnancy

1. Tighten the muscles of the pelvic floor.
2. Speak and see how the mouth, jaw and cheeks feel. This connection can be felt quite clearly if you try to tighten the pelvic floor and speak at the same time.

Techniques during contractions

Stop what you are doing, lean against your partner (or a wall) or lie down when the contraction starts.

1. Let your whole face relax and let your jaw go loose.
2. Relax your shoulders, let them sink down softly, lower and lower. Relax the rest of the body and let your arms, hands, tummy and backside sink down. Give yourself over to gravity.
3. Let the word 'heavy, heavy, heavy' vibrate inside.

FOCUS

In the midst of giving birth everything can seem chaotic. This is often expressed in frantic jerky movements of the body and eyes. By focusing the gaze on something specific you can ease the feeling of chaos which makes it easier to concentrate on relaxing and becoming heavy. I used a candle for my first birth, but anything works: a corner, a lamp, a picture or looking into someone's eyes.

WARMTH

Warmth creates security, calm and relaxation. The heat will help you to stay relaxed and in the flow. Hot water bottles, showers and baths are good pain reducers. If you take a bath drink some extra water to prevent dehydration, and place a cold, damp cloth over your head to stop yourself from feeling dizzy.

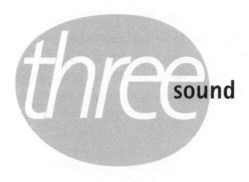
three sound

I am at Lotta and Filip's house working as a doula. The contractions have started with great force. Lotta is a little tense and I suggest she takes a bath. The warm water surrounds her body when she sinks down into the tub. She finds her breath and her weight, and she is able to relax. We keep working and the contractions come and go. The contractions get more and more intense and she is having trouble giving in to them, even though she is breathing soundlessly and relaxing her body. She is moving around restlessly in the bath. She can no longer remain calm during her contractions, and I see panic in her eyes. She works hard at relaxation, but I can see it is not helping her. It is like she is trying to hold a tornado back with her breathing. When I look at her body an image comes to mind. It is an image of something imploding and I realize I have to help her to let go of this force. During the contraction I ask her to use a sound. I can see that her body is trying to create a sound. Yes! These sounds will help her face the pain. Her body knows, but her fear stops her from realizing it. I lean in and whisper that her body wants something and that I will help her explore what that something is. I slowly guide her to let her exhalations grow into sound:

'Let the pain become a sound when you feel the rush. Open your mouth and make a deep sound all the way from below your navel. Flow with the energy of the body and make the sound deep. Good, that is great, keep going.'

She is slowly starting to greet the sensations with sound. Her voice grows darker and deeper. She is able to relax her jaw and get the sound from deep within. The bathroom vibrates from her deep sounds. She has found what she was looking for, something to help her through the pain. She stops fidgeting and she is able to sink down and remain relaxed. The difference is huge. Her contractions are strong and moving along. She keeps making sounds and her husband joins in. The acoustics in the bathroom amplify the noises and it sounds like a concert. She uses the sound during the second half of her delivery and it is also what helps her to push her beautiful baby out.

It can be very difficult to remain soundless during the last part of the delivery. The body is working hard and it is a very physical process. The pressure on the pelvic floor intensifies as the baby moves further down the birth canal. One way of assisting the body in this work is to make sounds. The body needs to release sounds. We use sounds to let go of what we are feeling. We laugh when we are happy, cry when we are sad, yell when we are angry, and use deep sounds and sighs when satisfied. This is a way of releasing some of the pressure. Many women feel the need to make sounds during labour. It is freeing and feels great! It can also help to let the physical aspect of your being take over. Making sounds is a good way to greet the pain during the latter part of labour. Even if a woman is embarrassed about making a noise, the physical impulse to do so during labour can be very intense. Try to see this as a natural part of delivery.

DEEP HEALING PITCH

Use a deep, dark tone. This will help you to stay relaxed and to fight off stress and fear. The deep, dark notes will engage the muscles in the pelvic floor, and help you bear down with the help of so-called intra-abdominal pressure. The muscles in the abdomen are arranged both vertically and horizontally. The muscles in the pelvic floor can be both relaxed and tight at the same time. All this is designed to let the baby travel slowly down the birth canal. By using the deep, dark sounds the body can be helped to slowly let the baby down.

In contrast, a forced high-pitched sound can invoke fear, which will increase muscle tightness and will in turn breed even more fear. This will block the body and put you in lockdown mode, causing a lot of valuable energy to get lost.

exercise

VOICE EXERCISES

Exercise during pregnancy

1. Lie or sit comfortably. Pay attention to your breathing as you have in previous exercises. Make a 'mmmm' sound with closed lips when you exhale. The sound should be even and last as long as you exhale. Repeat a few times.
2. Open your mouth. Relax your jaw and make a 'zzzzz' sound, then a 'ssss' sound. Repeat a few times. These consonants make great pushing sounds. Try to murmur or grumble. This might be just what you need to ease the pressure.
3. Relax your jaw and lips. Add more focus to each exhalation and use a deep 'aaahh' sound. Do not force the rhythm of your breathing, but use your own natural pace. Relax your shoulders.

▼

4. Play with making the sound darker and stronger. Can you feel your abdominal muscles when you make a dark sound?
5. Now explore how it makes you feel when using a high pitch and say 'eeeee' when you breathe out. What muscles are you activating? What happens in your throat? Where does the power go?
6. Go back to the dark, soft voice. Repeat a few times. What sensations can you feel? Can you feel the energy and direct it downwards through your system?

Technique during contractions

1. Use a deep dark voice as the contraction gets stronger. Relax the jaw, lips and throat. Extend the sound as long as you exhale.
2. The angle of the chin matters. If the chin is kept close to the chest, the throat area is locked. Lean the head back slightly and open up. Try what works and feels best for you.

Making sound

exercise

Keeping your head back slightly can help you to release the sound. Practise, especially if you are not used to making sounds like these. In this way you will be able to find what works best for you. Remember: what feels strange now might feel just right during labour.

1. Make the sound as in previous exercises.
2. Now, push the chin towards the chest and keep sounding. Repeat a few times.
3. Lean the head back slightly. Let the sound emerge through soft lips, and keep the palms of the hands open. How does it feel? Repeat a few times.

SOUND AND BREATHING

You can use the sound as a technique both to welcome the contractions at the end of delivery as well as to help push the baby out. The sound can help to maintain a soft and steady rhythm of breathing since it is often difficult to prolong your exhalations in the final phase of delivery. The sounds are simply used as exhalations, and are repeated over and over again. Remember to keep the sound soft and not too high.

When the sound is used as a pushing technique, the woman can flow with the pressure while activating the abdominal muscles.

the power of the mind

As I start my shift as an assistant nurse I walk into the room of a second-time mother. She is about to start pushing. I have read in her birth plan that she is afraid this birth is going to be a repeat of her previous labour. Everything had moved along fine until she entered the pushing phase when she completely shut down. They ended up having to use forceps and she did not want that to happen again. I observe her for a while. I can see how her body is readjusting as it prepares for the pushing phase. As I stand watching her I can see how her body literally shuts down. It gets tense and starts pulling upwards. Her face, neck, thighs and jaw are rigid and tense. I try to help her with my tools, but to no avail. I realize that she is facing what she fears the most. Time passes and the body is not able to access its power even though it tries. She is fighting hard to gain control, but it doesn't work. She is almost out of time by now. The staff are preparing the vacuum extractor. I am desperate because I want to help her, but I don't know how. I have another tool that I haven't presented to her yet – to say the word 'yes'. But where am I going to get the courage to tell someone I have only met for an hour that it can work to simply 'say yes'? She is probably going to ask me to get out of the room. To simply say 'yes' at a time like this seems a little crazy, but I decide to take a chance.

While the forceps are being prepared I lean in towards her. 'You are going to think I am a fool, but I have a suggestion to help you dare to push. Would you try it for three contractions?' She looks at me like I am a crazy person, but agrees to try – she is willing to try anything at this point. When the contraction rolls in she utters a weak 'yesss'. I praise her, but I realize she needs more power to be able to use this tool to its full potential. I encourage her to try again, but this time with her mouth wide open. When the next contraction comes I say 'yes' with her. She opens her mouth slowly and a strong and resolute 'yeeeeeeeeeeeeeeeees' emerges. This sound springs from deep within her. Her body moves and a few seconds later her baby arrives. The midwife and the obstetrician are puzzled and the woman is dazed. I stand there in amazement. The woman is overjoyed! She looks up at me. 'That was so strange. It felt like a string that just snapped! The muscles relaxed and just let the baby go. Thank you!' I stood there amazed and grateful, and I realized I had found an incredibly powerful tool.

I will never forget the first day I used this tool. It was crucial for my understanding of the power of the human mind. Since that day I have used this tool during many deliveries and it is one of my most powerful tools.

SAY 'YES'

Saying 'yes' is just one of many different ways to access your inner power. Thoughts are very powerful and can be used in many ways. People working in the cognitive psychology field have known this for many years. You can unlock every mental blockage using a positive thought. During a contraction you can use the word 'down' if you feel like you are having a hard time flowing along with your body. This thought will send signals to your muscles causing them to release and let go. To allow yourself to be calm during pain, you can say, 'open' as a reminder of where to focus your energy. If you start saying 'no', just do the opposite and say 'yes'. You can move mountains by the sheer force of your mind!

When overwhelmed by pain, it is easy to say 'no'. This is automatic when you are taken by surprise. Sometimes you do not even notice and it is impossible to do anything else. However, it is more important than ever to say 'yes' when the feelings are negative. It sounds stupid, crazy, and maybe even insane, but the word 'yes' directly engages parts of the brain to find positive emotions, faith and power. This is an effect of expectations. By saying the word 'yes' you put the body in a place where it will not lock down. Neurologically it is unbeatable!

This mind tool magically influences the inner motivation to withstand the pain, and helps you to cope with labour. The word 'yes' helps you to accept and have faith in what happens. This is very important when facing the force and power of birth, and is neurologically unbeatable. It is similar to the way the body says 'yes' when it feels safe (the peace and calm system), and the body's 'no' response to stress and fear (the stress system). By saying the word 'yes' you stimulate even more power and confidence both mentally and physiologically.

You can choose only to use the physical tools we have talked about when facing your contractions. You will find them very valuable. This can be a difficult tool to use if you are not comfortable doing something that might feel a little crazy. It can, however, be a very powerful tool if you choose to use it.

Many women wonder when to start using this tool. The answer is simple: use it when you start to feel the urge to say 'no', 'I can't take it' or 'I do not want this'. If you are going to say something, say 'yes'. This is a much better way to welcome the baby. Often women who start saying 'yes' keep doing so for many hours. Many obstetricians tend to look a little confused when hearing this mantra of 'yes, yes, yes' for hours.

Technique during pregnancy

To really understand the close relationship between words and the body, try the following exercises.

Nod/shake your head

1. Nod as you say 'yes'. Repeat a few times.
2. Shake your head as you say 'yes'. Repeat a few times.

To say 'yes/no'
1. Put the book away and relax your jaw, shoulders, arms, hips and legs.
2. In silence think 'yes' and then 'no'. Let the word vibrate inside your head. Repeat a few times. Did it feel different?
3. Let your exhalations turn into a deep sound. Repeat a few times. Open your mouth wide and let the deep sound turn into a 'yes' said with a nice dark tone. Let the sound be as long as your exhalation. Repeat a few times. How did that feel?
4. Now say 'noooooo'. Repeat a few times. What was the difference? How did that feel?
5. Go back to slowly saying 'yeeeees' with an open, relaxed mouth, using your deep voice. Let the head fall back just a little bit as you speak.

Technique during contractions

1. Softly, with a deep voice say 'yeeees' using a rhythm that is comfortable.
2. Tilt your head back slightly if that feels comfortable. This posture helps you to stay open. Do what feels best for you.

MANTRA

Find a mantra that works for you. It may not be the word 'yes'. You might want to use the name of your partner or the word 'down'. A mantra helps to keep worry at bay. It also reduces the activity level in the brain by keeping it occupied. When your mind is unable to create worry, it releases the 'feel good' hormone oxytocin. Do not be afraid to try this during labour, even if you do not expect it to work. The technique that is most effective during labour is sometimes the one you might least have expected to work. Use what you learned when reading about the previous tool (sound). Make the sound into a word. I have heard women using nothing but the sound tool throughout the whole latent part of the birthing process. The sound is like a mantra that you can focus on.

Suggestions on words to use as a mantra:
- Yes
- Down
- A name, maybe your partner's
- My baby
- Open

AFFIRMATIONS

Thoughts are the foundations of life. They can either get in the way, or they can be used to help. The thoughts come from you, and therefore you have all the power to change the ones that get in your way. When you consciously redirect your thoughts to take a more positive course, you are using affirmations. Negative thoughts can be exchanged for positive ones. If you keep repeating an uplifting positive thought the subconsciousness will recognize it as the 'truth'. In this way you can mobilize your own healing powers. Your body will use this new 'truth' without questioning if it is 'real' or 'made up'.

Affirmations that work are positive and stated in the present tense. Do not use the word 'never' in your affirmations.

Affirmations

Only use affirmations that will strengthen you. Deliberately use positive thoughts in place of negative ones. This is what affirmations are all about. Use affirmations throughout your pregnancy. Write them down in a notebook and keep it next to your bed. Repeat the affirmations a few times in the morning and again at night. Reinforce the positive expectation by actively building faith and trust.

- I am strong and calm.
- I trust my body.
- I can handle the pain.
- I understand I am afraid, but I can handle it.
- I accept all my feelings.

exercise

VISUALIZING

Imagine your breath as a waterfall. This will help you to move in the same direction as your body. You are visualizing. You can picture how the pain opens the door for the baby, or that you are in a place where you feel safe and cozy. The effect you get when visualizing is similar to the effect you get when using affirmations. Emotions connected to these pictures will help you to break fear and stress.

I was attending a birth where the pushing phase was difficult. The labouring woman was not aware of how much she was tensing up. The midwife saw that the woman's pelvic floor was white and tight due to the lack of blood flow. We started working with her breathing to help her relax and to increase circulation. I instructed her to imagine how the inhalation came from a place above her head, and how the exhalation ran through her like a waterfall, through her chest and belly and out through her pelvic floor. Breath by breath we worked and she eventually found a rhythm and a way to picture this waterfall inside of her. Ten minutes after we started, her pelvic floor was elastic and pliable. By using her mind she had come in contact with the sublime tension in her pelvis. The midwife and I witnessed this transformation in amazement.

exercise

Technique during contractions
1. Visualize your inhalation coming from a place above your head.
2. Imagine your exhalation as a waterfall, which softly and quietly runs through your chest, belly and pelvis. Repeat several times at your own pace.

Using the tools during labour

LATENCY PHASE

You might not need any of the tools during the latency phase. It may be enough to listen to your breathing and check to see if you are relaxed during the rush. Your support person does not need to work very hard at this point in the process, since you are probably capable of relaxing and going with the flow as the contractions come and go.

It is important, however, that the beginning of childbirth is good, and that you are able to relax when you need to. Some women can have an intense and painful experience in this phase. They will need the support person to be an active participant from the beginning. Use all your senses when deciding what support is needed at any given time. Remember to conserve your mental capacity by distracting yourself.

DURING THE OPENING PHASE

You are now using the tools more and more, and this requires a great deal of concentration. During each contraction use the four tools to sink down and welcome the contraction, allowing the body to do its job. The present is the only thing that matters. Try not to think about the coming contraction. At the start of this phase you might not need the support person that much. As the contractions take you further and further, you will feel an increasing need for the support of your partner.

When you are six to ten centimetres dilated at the end of the opening phase you might have a hard time breathing softly and calmly. This is when you can use your voice as a guide to keep the rhythm. This is also when a lot of women start saying 'no'. They do not want to participate any longer and fear begins to take over. They may feel like they will not be able to handle the situation, which creates a sense of hopelessness. This is the time when the mental tool of saying 'yes' is very important. It is a very effective way to turn the negative thoughts around, and open up the mind to the idea of daring to give birth.

DURING PUSHING

Keep using the four tools while in the pushing phase. Emphasize the feeling of heaviness. It is helpful to sink down towards your heels while kneeling when you need to push. The most important thing is to maintain the downward movement, letting the body sink towards the floor. Bend your knees if you are standing upright. If your legs are tired you can lie down on your side, but keep your mind focused on sinking down. Think or say the word 'down'. It is as if you are coaching the baby deep inside to go 'down, down, down you go'. Do this while your buttocks sink down towards your heels.

If you vocalize you have a powerful tool with which to greet the contraction. Keep the sound deep and even. It is not a scream. If you use this technique while pushing you might need to close your lips at the end. This creates an 'mmm' sound, directing all the power down through your body.

Women frequently lock themselves in a certain pattern during this phase. It can feel impossible to break free from this behaviour. If this is true for you, try using the word 'yes'. The word 'yes' has an almost magical ability to unlock barriers and open up the experience.

PUSHING TECHNIQUE

There is a tendency to panic when it gets to the pushing phase. It is easy to get swept up in all the cheering and pushing. It might sound unbelievable, but it is possible to be calm during this phase. Many women need time to be able to let go enough and find the courage to let the baby out. The muscles in the pelvic floor need to be relaxed for the baby to pass. If the pelvic floor is tightened while bearing down, two strong forces are working against each other. Picture the muscles of the uterus pushing from above while the baby, head first, jostles down through the soft relaxed tissue of the pelvis. There are no obstacles or tension in the way. This image might work for you during this phase.

You do not have to bear down for all you are worth. You should be completely passive until you can no longer resist pushing. You run the risk of unconsciously pushing too hard if you feel overtaken by the force of the contractions. It might feel as if pushing is the only thing you can do. But the fact is that you have to be able to resist pushing, while not resisting the movement inside. Do not go along with the forced feeling you might get when you feel the impulse to bear down. Remain in the moment and take in how it feels if you remain passive. In this way you create a connection with the body's impulse to bear down. You also allow the tissues time to soften and stretch.

If the pushing contractions are weak it might be difficult to find the right muscles. Weak contractions in this phase can be due to a tired uterus, pain medications or there might be something else. The midwife will help you to find a technique that can work for you and allow you to find a strong inner force. If the contractions are strong, there is nothing to worry about.

For the pelvic floor to be able to relax you can use the movement and direction of your breathing. Focus on exhaling through your chest, stomach and pelvis. This has done miracles in many of the births I have attended. Using the deep, dark voice or a murmur also has this magical effect and can help you to softly flow in tune with the birth process. Dare to find your own way.

exercise

Finding the right muscles

What you need to do during the pushing phase is to find the right muscles in your pelvic floor, and the pressure in your abdominals, the intra-abdominal pressure. Below are a few exercises for you to practise finding your muscles, and to get a feeling for what it is like to bear down.

1. Use the deep voice. Close your mouth and feel the sound inside the chest and mouth. Repeat a few times and see how it feels.
2. Imagine you have to push a tampon out of the vagina. Do not use the same muscles as when you are having a bowel movement. Try a few times and reflect on the sensation.
3. A fun exercise to do, and one that works remarkably well, is to arm wrestle. When you are trying to get your partner's arm down you are using the muscles you need to push the baby out. Do this a few times and take some time to reflect. Try doing it again, now adding the deep voice. Didn't that work much better? Try closing your mouth and direct the sound down towards your pelvis.
4. Do the same thing using the murmur technique. This will help you not to overdo it while pushing.

Movement and rest during labour

To facilitate the birth process you need to shift gears every so often between activity and rest. The upright activities of walking, hip rotation and changing positions during birth will promote increased blood circulation, stimulate the contractions and help the baby move down through the birth canal. Use the four tools during the contractions as well as the other techniques we have discussed.

It can be a good idea to bring along some music. The music you find most helpful might not be in the style you had anticipated. I was attending a birth where the labouring mother had brought some soothing melodies with dolphin sounds. When we turned it on the woman got angry and yelled at us to turn it off. It turned out the music did not match at all what she was feeling through the pain and contractions. She asked us to turn on the radio instead. By sheer chance Michael Jackson's *Bad* was playing. The mother-to-be instinctively started moving her hips in rhythm with the music. It looked quite comical and we all broke out in a big laugh. Laughing through her pain she exclaimed how this music better corresponded with what she needed.

Movements that can work during the active phases:
- Walking or wandering around.
- Circling and moving the hips while thinking 'heavy, heavy' or some other mantra.
- Stand upright or keep changing position.
- In the event you have had an epidural, it is important for you to keep moving around to stimulate contractions so that they do not stop. You will be able to move around even though you have taken an epidural.

MOVE THE HIPS

Softly and rhythmically move the hips around during the rushes. The movement releases tension and can give you a lovely feeling. I once heard a midwife give a good description of the benefits of this action. 'Imagine you have a ring on your finger', she said. 'To get this ring off you need to fold, bend and twist your finger while pulling the ring towards you. This is exactly the way the baby needs to be moved down in your pelvis.' It is also nice to 'do' something with the pain and through the action feel some sense of power. You are participating and the movement is your guide. Swing from side to side or move like a belly dancer. Let your head be slightly tilted back. This opens the jaw and helps you to relax the pelvic floor muscles. Try out different movements and positions. Use the four tools and the thought of being heavy while exploring the movements.

Stand upright or use gravity to facilitate the work the body needs to do. It does not mean you have to stand upright throughout the entire birth, but try to avoid lying on your back as much as possible. Few women choose to lie on their back during childbirth. Most women instinctively know it will make the process more difficult, both for accessing their own inner power, and using the physical laws of gravity. Lying flat on the back instantly makes it anatomically like working uphill, and the circulation to the uterus decreases. Try to find upright positions, or at least try sitting up if you have to be on your back.

REST

It is early in the morning and I am on my way to the hospital to attend the birth of Janet and Thomas's baby. Two wrecks greet me as I enter the room. Neither of them has slept in two days, and Janet is having a hard time with the contractions. She is dejected. Thomas is literally breaking down right in front of my eyes. He is terrified he won't be able to be the solid support she needs and the thought makes him distressed. I quickly decide they need to sleep. I close the curtains and turn the light off. Gently, I get them to lie down, head to head, on two beanbags. Slowly I guide them towards a calm, soft and soundless breathing. I encourage them to give in and let go of all control. 'You do not have to do anything right now. Give in. Surrender. Everything is alright.'

The first little twitch comes soon afterwards. I keep speaking using a deep, calm voice. Another twitch, then I hear deep breathing. They are both asleep. They were finally able to let go and the much longed for rest could come. Janet wakes up during each contraction, but is able to go right back to sleep as soon as the rush has subsided. After 45 minutes they wake up refreshed. They are fascinated and surprised. They never thought they would be able to fall asleep, or that resting would be so valuable.

We keep working actively throughout the day. Janet is using the tools during each rush. The birth process is moving along slowly and she is not opening up very much. By the end of the afternoon she is exhausted and I am able to help her rest once again. She gives in completely and quickly falls into a deep sleep. Suddenly, while sleeping she starts opening up in a furious rush. Since she is not afraid, she keeps sleeping between the contractions.

She sits up during each rush, looks at Thomas and me and says, 'No... epidural.' We understand this to be more of a question. Will I be able to handle this? We put our hands on her. 'It is okay. Everything is okay. Let go... heavy... heavy... heavy.'

Her whole body relaxes and she falls back to sleep. The next contraction rolls in after about 30 seconds.

'No epidural.'

We calmly respond and put our hands on her body. She sinks down, tilts back and falls asleep once again. We keep this routine going for the next 40 minutes. After approximately 40 minutes she starts to sense the urge to bear down. We understand she is almost completely open by now. She gets down on a mattress on the floor and crouches on all fours. Recharged with new energy she uses the deep voice to be able to keep up with the pushing impulses. Aided by the soft instructions from her midwife and the support from her husband she peacefully pushes her baby out.

It sounds unbelievable, but it is possible to sleep during active labour. In a prolonged birth process sleep is one of the most important components. The midwife Cayenne Ekjordh taught me this when I worked with her as an assistant nurse. Her 'diving technique' helps women relax to the point of being able to sleep all the way through the pushing phase. I have been inspired to help women relax and sleep during their labour ever since I learned this technique.

Both the body and the mind need time to recover if the woman is going to have the stamina to last all through a long birth. No technique or tool in the world can be a help to you if you do not get to rest and recover between rushes.

Some labours are quick and there is no need to sleep. More often, though, childbirth takes time, especially if it is the woman's first baby. Sleep is important for the hormonal system, and has a restorative function. Most importantly, sleep is essential for mental stamina, which will help the woman to bond with her newborn. Mental strength is also important when it comes to keeping negative thoughts from taking over.

If the mind does not get any rest there is a risk that the woman will develop symptoms of stress, such as lethargy, anxiety and resignation. These feelings can cloud her from seeing the significance of what happens, and lead to a negative view of the birth experience. No human being is able to stay awake for more than 24 hours without developing some feelings of anxiety. Insomnia is by no means part of the process of childbirth.

Obviously, you are not meant to snore your way through the entire labour, but you should be able to take power naps between the contractions. The sleep I am talking about is not uninterrupted, but rather a state that sets in between each rush. As the contractions come with shorter and shorter intervals it might be uncomfortable to wake up every time a contraction comes, but it is still a resting period for your body to enjoy.

SLEEP DURING CHILDBIRTH

Sleep is at the opposite end of the spectrum from fear and stress. You will only be able to relax enough to fall asleep if you are feeling safe, and have faith in the fact that what you are going through is not harmful in any way. If you use the technique of letting the body become heavy and completely relaxed between the contractions the body will sense how you are letting go of control. This is a signal that resting and sleeping is permitted.

You need to cease talking between the contractions to be able to fall asleep. Try to let go of the thinking mind. Dare to stay in a relaxed mood during, and in between contractions, since this will open up the possibility of falling asleep. You will need a great deal of courage to do this, but keep in mind that it will not make the contractions harder. It will only make it easier for you to fall back to sleep when the rush subsides.

Technique:

- Turn off the lights and make the room dark.
- Find a position where the head, neck and shoulders are relaxed. You might want to lie on your side or be half sitting.
- The support person can give you a hand or foot massage. The movement should be rhythmical, calm and monotonous. Keep massaging the same place over and over.
- During the massage the support person can repeat a word or a sentence using a slow, soft, deep voice. Try one of a few words like 'heavy', 'relax' or 'let go'. The continuous motion of the massage and the mantra will diminish the brain's ability to register pain. A trance-like state will set in.

We are focusing on short little power naps in between contractions. It can take 20 minutes until you are relaxed enough, but keep massaging, be quiet and keep the room dark. When you feel as though you have regained some strength you can work actively again for a few hours. I have seen a pattern emerge, where most awake periods last for between four and six hours, and most sleep periods are about 40 to 90 minutes in length. A sleep period is followed by an active period. Women who have faith in their bodies and the birth process sometimes fall asleep for short periods while sitting or standing.

Resting and recuperating are also important for the support person. I am not suggesting that he or she should sleep for several hours (unless of course that is okay for you), but rather that he or she gets shorter periods of rest in order to provide the best possible support.

3

Support and confidence

During the years I have worked as a doula I have come to understand how important the support person is for a woman in labour. This chapter is therefore aimed both at the mother and the support person. The support person has a key role to play in preventing worry and fear during birth. Continuous support during labour has been proven to decrease the likelihood of a Caesarean section, shorten the process, and, most importantly, give the woman a positive birth experience. The support person is the anchor in a stormy sea with waves of contractions and will give you faith and stamina when yours are failing. The support person is also the one to make you aware of the physical reactions created by fear and stress. Therefore it is very important for the support person to prepare for the delivery. Preparing together will give the support person the confidence to guide you through the birth process, and it will give you the faith to follow along.

Giving support

Supporting a woman in labour is not always an easy task. During the birthing process she will temporarily leave the world you normally share. She will enter into a sphere where her body takes over. Your support is crucial for her when that happens. By knowing how a birth normally proceeds you will be able to help her stay calm and in the natural flow of labour.

Most people experience labour as an unfamiliar event. You cannot automatically be expected to know what needs to be done if you haven't been given information beforehand. This chapter will help you to be a better support for the labouring woman. It will give some practical advice, for example, on how to use the most valuable tools a support person will need – massage and touch. You can read and use this entire book, or you can use this chapter only. My wish is to inspire you to trust yourself. Your love and presence is what counts.

It is a calm evening in June and I am out on a doula mission. Fredrik opens the door for me. Petra is in the bathroom, on the toilet. I walk into the bathroom and make sure to establish body contact with her. We instantly connect. I look into her misty eyes. I observe her for a moment, and I see how she has trouble focusing her eyes. I see how her body is uneasy and I can hear her breathing. I whisper that I am there to support her. Using a deep, slow voice I start to explain what is happening in her body, how her body is working downwards and how she just needs to follow along by becoming heavy during the contractions. Through the contractions I remind her to get heavy and breathe quietly. I encourage her to relax her jaw and her shoulders and to dare to be heavy. By helping her to focus her eyes I get her to stay in the moment. I soon feel how she gets heavier and how she lets go. Her body is working with the contractions. Everything is moving along well and Petra stands up, supporting herself on Fredrik and me. Fredrik massages and rubs her back with downward movements to help her let go even more.

In this posture, the contractions seem to intensify and become more powerful. Petra bends her legs and follows the direction of the baby. After each contraction we help her to fill her lungs and to sigh softly. The contractions get increasingly more forceful and soon the tools are not enough for her. It gets harder and harder for her to flow and work downwards. She keeps repeating how tired she is and how it will not work. In spite of all this, she keeps breathing softly and her body is heavy. She is helping her body, but mentally it is more difficult. I encourage Fredrik to move closer and whisper in her ear: 'I am here for you... you can do it... I am here for you... follow the movement... let go... I am here.'

They are standing very close together and he is right there for her. I can see how quickly he picks up on what she needs. He knows exactly how to talk to her and he is protecting her. Using a deep voice he guides her through the contractions. The midwife and I are there to support the two of them. They only need us when the labour moves into a new phase, but mostly they want to be alone.

Petra starts getting the urge to push. As a team we guide her to move with the direction of the pressure, and to find her deep tone. She finds a pitch that works for her and her bottom starts to move towards the floor.

The baby moves further down the birth canal after each contraction. By being fully present in the moment she is able to let her body work at its own pace. There are several cries of 'no' and 'I can't do this!' during the process. She needs to be able to express these emotions and we support her. It is time. Petra feels the head and I will always remember her eyes, filled *with wonder and gratitude. With each rush the baby's head moves closer and closer to the opening. Petra is ready to release the baby into the room. It is quiet and calm. Petra suddenly stands up and the head emerges. Soon a baby boy is born.*

CHOOSING A SUPPORT PERSON

Having a support person during labour is very important. Security and support will help keep negative emotions away. The labouring woman needs to feel seen and respected during the whole process. She might end up feeling alone even though there are people in the room. Often this is because the people around her are unaware of how to help.

Carefully consider what kind of support the pregnant woman would like to have. If you are the woman's partner you are the most important support. You can either choose to be the sole support person, if you are comfortable with that, or you can choose to share the task with someone close to the woman, or a doula. Having an extra person present doesn't imply the woman considers her partner to be inept. The doula's task is to help create a positive birth experience for the two of you. If the pregnant woman does not want to bring a partner to the delivery room, having a doula is a good alternative.

DOULA

A doula is a woman who is professionally trained to assist women before, during and after childbirth. She gives the labouring woman, and her partner, continuous physical, emotional and informational support. The word doula comes from a Greek word meaning 'a woman who serves'. Throughout history experienced women have been part of childbirth. When deliveries started to take place in hospitals instead of in the home, important support for the labouring woman was forgotten.

Giving birth is safer than ever today, but at the same time it can also be more stressful and lonelier than ever. The main task of the doula is to protect the birth experience and to guide the labouring woman and her partner by sharing useful tools and techniques for facing the challenges ahead. She supports the woman in whatever decision she makes. A doula respects the fact that all women are different and have different needs. Her task is also to nurture the women through her contractions by using massage, touch and emotional support. As a doula she does not belong to a specific clinic, neither does she have any medical role in the delivery process. She is not a substitute for a midwife. She does not usually have a medical degree. Her role consists of nurturing the labouring woman and her partner throughout the labour, however long it might last. She can focus on encouraging and comforting, without having to worry about anything else.

There are many active doulas working today. Some of them work professionally and others on a voluntary basis. There are companies and organizations that facilitate contacts between women and doulas. For more details see page 188.

Massage and touch

When the birthing woman first encounters pain her brain reacts by trying to understand and control the sensations. She tries to take charge with her mind and to control the next contraction, how long it will last, the level of pain and how long the labour will go on. The brain is working frantically and a lot of energy is wasted. Since the intellect is not able to give birth, it gets in the way of the body accessing its own intelligence. One way of interrupting mental activity is by touch or closeness. Touch will pull the energy from the brain to the body. The birthing woman will feel heavy and tired, she will feel a greater connection with her own body and her mind will quieten down. She can slowly relax, forgetting about time and space, and focusing only on the present. She does not care about what happens outside, and is able to settle serenely into her body. Talk, thoughts and control lose their grip and she is able to surf on the waves of the rushes.

These are the reasons massage and touch are such powerful tools for the support person to have. The skin is our biggest sensory organ. Massage can be a wonderful way of stimulating strength and inner power. Touch releases the body's pain-relieving substances, which will bring calm, tranquillity and a chance to recover. Through massage and touch the support person is able to communicate directly with the body of the labouring woman. By using your hands you can feel if her body is tense or relaxed, and there is no need for words.

I am assisting Cina and Joel as a doula. When I arrive I find Cina all revved up in full motion. She is almost running round in circles, and is surprised by the pace and force of the contractions. The fight-or-flight behaviour is obvious. She is constantly moving, her muscles are tense, her gaze keeps shifting and her motions are jerky. I approach and make body contact with her. I softly caress her and make her lean on me, with her head resting on my shoulder. She immediately shifts to a lower gear. We are standing really close to each other, swaying back and forth through a few contractions. The rhythm is slow and soothing and she is resting, letting the rushes come and go. When we have found the rhythm, and she has landed in her body, her husband Joel takes over. They are standing close together for a long time. She feels completely safe and present in the moment. The closeness helps her to relax, and time keeps moving forward. After a while she wants to lie on her side of the bed. She is heavy and brave and is able to breathe deeply. In spite of this she has a hard time trying not to tense up. We start massaging her by pulling our hands from her shoulders, down her back and down to her hips. It relaxes her enough and she is able to rest for a while.

The contractions are becoming more and more forceful. She works on breathing soundlessly, and feeling heavy. We keep massaging her to be able to be in the moment. The midwife arrives and joins us. Joel is right there, close to his wife, massaging and caressing her, encouraging her, and showing her that he is right there for her. She has body contact all the time and the massages keep her calm and serene. We can hear it's time to push and so we help her down onto some pillows on the floor. Her husband is encouraging her, guiding her along, and she is able to follow. Soon the head of the baby is visible. Cina is completely relaxed and able to rest between pushes. Her body is able to recharge and have energy to push the baby out. A beautiful girl is born and the mood is calm.

Oxytocin

Massage works because of the positive effect of oxytocin. As we saw in Chapter 1, oxytocin is one of the hormones involved in directing the contractions and in the mechanism of breastfeeding. Oxytocin is released by touch, heat, safety and calm. It is often called the 'calm and tranquillity hormone'. Oxytocin counteracts fear and stress, and has a noticeable effect on reducing anxiety. It can help the woman to relax, or fall asleep momentarily during childbirth.

Most importantly, oxytocin has the power to lessen pain. The pain is still present and is registered, but it is not felt as strongly and does not seem so frightening. Oxytocin also helps the mother bond with her child, and it makes the attachment stronger and more immediate.

Gate control theory

Massage can also work through the 'gate control theory'. This theory is based upon the fact that the sensations from touch and pain take different paths to the brain. If these impulses arrive at the same time, the pain impulses are overridden by the touch impulses by means of a mechanism that gives priority to the touch impulses. The brain perceives a smaller number of pain impulses, and therefore the woman experiences less pain.

MASSAGE DURING CONTRACTIONS

Oxytocin is released by a 'nice' touch, closeness and comfortable warmth. Therefore classic massage might not be the most comfortable as it usually goes deep into the muscle tissue. You should try to stroke, squeeze gently and use a light touch. This is known as the pleasure massage or the tactile massage. Always massage from the head down, since this reinforces the direction of the contractions and the downward movement of the baby.

Flowing massage

TECHNIQUE DURING CONTRACTIONS: Use an open palm and keep the fingers straight and slightly apart. The support person uses the entire hand (but with emphasis on the fingers) along the back and arms. The movement is one long sweep and with a strong firm pressure.

Squeeze massage

TECHNIQUE DURING CONTRACTIONS: Keep your fingers together and your hand slightly cupped as if you are squeezing a snowball. Start massaging the neck and move down the arms and shoulders, down the back and towards the hips, buttocks and thighs. Squeeze, let go, squeeze, let go.

Butterfly massage

If the pain is strong around the groins and pubic bone, the support person can apply a technique called the butterfly massage. This involves a very light touch, like the wings of a butterfly, to the groin area, the stomach and any other place on the birthing mother's body. The butterfly massage works as a pain inhibitor since it distracts the pain.

TECHNIQUE DURING CONTRACTIONS: Use your fingers to make light sweeping butterfly movements over the stomach and groins.

A labouring woman can do this by herself by standing up, and swaying from side to side while tickling her own belly. It is soothing, and the tickling will distract the pain impulses. Try helping her by making sweeping butterfly movements with your fingers over her belly and groin. The pain can sometimes be particularly intense in the groin. The butterfly massage will relieve some of this pain. Try using your nails lightly, and then try without using your nails.

Firm pressure on the lumbar region

As the labour progresses the pain will move from the groin to the lumbar area, or the lower back. The butterfly massage works very well in the groin, but the back needs more force. The strong sensation in the back can also be present from the beginning of labour.

TECHNIQUE DURING CONTRACTIONS: By circling the base of your hands over her lower back the pain impulses are blocked. Make the circles small and firm.

In case you do not find any of these techniques helpful you can always invent your own massage technique. Remember to focus on the movement and work from the top of the body, down along the arms, back, hips and legs.

STAY CLOSE

In our everyday lives we have a circle of approximately one metre as our private sphere. We usually wish to keep strangers out of this space. A birthing woman does not usually need to keep this distance. Instead she is open to, and in need of closeness, support and touch. The closeness helps her to be brave and give in to the birthing process. It feels good to snuggle up close to someone. It feels safe, and she can relax in an organic and natural way. Negative emotions are less likely to take over while she is in body contact with someone. Closeness is comforting and makes her feel safe. While completely vulnerable and open to the experiences she might still feel short of energy and lacking in willpower. It means her sense of security is stronger than her fear. These feelings may co-exist, but the sense of safety the woman gets from the support person will help her to slowly move through the birth.

Crying or strong emotions are common during certain phases of childbirth. Remain in body contact with each other throughout the birth. This can be an amazing process that will make your bond stronger and your relationship richer and fuller. A woman can be close to her support person even though she is using laughing gas or has taken an epidural.

Exercise during pregnancy

1. Curl up on the bed or sofa.
2. Embrace the woman and make sure she is completely relaxed.
3. Try to keep close together with as much body contact as possible.
4. Practise to see how many parts of the body can be touched at any given time.
5. Explore what feels comfortable and good.

INSPIRATION

Get close to each other. Embrace her, hug and keep body contact. Show her it is okay to be open and vulnerable. Stand with your body facing the woman so that she feels completely safe and surrounded. Rock and sway during the rushes. This promotes security and relaxation. It is important to sway softly, calmly and slowly. Picking a fast rhythm will have the opposite effect and is a common mistake. The woman can also sway and rock by herself. I have observed many women while they sway from side to side, massaging their belly with eyes closed and completely wrapped up in their body.

Body contact will release oxytocin, and closeness helps the woman rest during the short breaks between contractions. Even the shortest breaks can be useful. If she feels safe and calm, she can use the breaks to fall asleep and regain her strength. Many people forget that it is okay to kiss during childbirth. Kissing keeps the jaw and mouth relaxed.

Some women feel uncomfortable and suffocated by closeness. If this is the case, you will have to guide her with words.

Guidelines for the support person

A woman in labour will commonly not be able to talk very much. Nor should she be expected to do so. Being quiet and turning inwards are ways for her to stay in touch with her body, and to focus on the physical work. Therefore it is important to find other ways to communicate, such as physical closeness, touch and signs or gestures.

DO NOT BE AFRAID OF HER PAIN

Witnessing someone you love and care for in great pain can trigger a lot of emotions and feelings in your own body. You might get the urge to call in the doctor and to inject her with every pain medication possible. Another possible scenario is that you will get stressed, because you don't know how to help her. Do not be afraid of her pain. She will need you to be strong and support her more than ever before. Right there in the eye of the storm it is crucial that you are able to take charge for a while and help her to stay steady. You might have to do this even though she says she can't stand it any more. It does not necessarily mean that she has given up when she says these things. She might just need to vent her frustration. It sometimes feels good for her to say that she does not want to continue any more, or that she wants drugs. In this instance she needs people around her to confirm what she is feeling and help her to get back on track.

She might become aggressive, be hard to communicate with or pull away in the process. You have to be there for her regardless of what happens. You have to trust your abilities and have faith in your role as a support person. Try not to take what happens personally. You are her most important guide.

DARE TO TAKE OVER IF SHE GETS LOST

The woman's body signals clearly when she is in a negative pattern. If you learn to read the body and its signals during stress you can help the labouring woman break the pattern she is in with the help of the tools. Be brave and dare to take over if you see her getting lost or losing focus. Finding the courage to assist someone who is stressed, lost or angry can be a lot harder than you think. It is a great challenge and it takes courage. You need to be able to express yourself clearly and confidently or the woman will not follow your advice. The guidelines in this chapter are meant to be a framework for you to work with, so that you can make suggestions while feeling secure and grounded in yourself. You will develop techniques so that you don't feel you are disturbing or interfering with the birth process. This will also allow the woman to feel free to choose whether or not she wants support or if she wants to use the tools. You are never meant to say 'Do this!' or 'Do that!' It is important that you stay sensitive to her needs.

DARE TO HELP

It can be difficult to know when, or how to intervene during labour. How firm should you be? What assistance should you offer? How should you act if she cries? What if she resists your help? The labouring woman will need you the most when she feels her power is lacking or that she is losing her momentum. This is when you have to step in. She needs you to lovingly take over and act as her source of power and faith. She needs to hear 'You can do this', 'I am here with you' and 'I will help you get through the next rush'. To prevent you from standing back in what you might think is respect while she is struggling, you need to come up with a plan in advance as to how to handle these situations. Agree on how she wants you to guide her even when she is mad, upset or frustrated. When, and if, she reaches an inner limit, you both need to be clear on how she can communicate this in a direct and easy way.

CREATE A SECURE ENVIRONMENT

The labouring woman needs you as a guide, coach and companion. You also have to create secure and safe surroundings for her. Fear will make her body close up and make the birth process stall. You need to help her to let go and flow with the body, regardless of whether or not she is using pain medication. Your task is to keep an eye on everything surrounding her so that she can focus on what is happening inside of her. This includes body contact, eye contact, light, sound and everything in your environment. Do not underestimate the importance of the surroundings.

STAY CLOSE

Stay physically close to the labouring woman during her contractions. Maintain body contact, and look her in the eyes when giving her instructions. This will keep her safe and make her feel secure. I heard of a woman who got a 'contraction storm'. This is when the uterus cramps and the contractions come without a break in between. The woman panicked. The pain was unbearable. Her husband did not know what to do. His instincts made him climb up on top of her and cradle her. This proved to be just what she needed. To her it felt like he was holding her together when her body threatened to break into a thousand pieces. Before her labour, she would have thought this sounded crazy, but at the time it was the only thing that worked. However, some women might need a lot of space. Most labouring women want closeness, but others do not. Everybody is different. Ask what feels right.

FIRM HANDS WITH RHYTHM

You need to be aware of how to touch the labouring woman. Using the tools calls for total awareness. A flimsy grip might be perceived as irritating or annoying. Use firm hands and gestures. Do not hesitate or be unclear in your movements. Let the touch be firm and strong. Rhythm is another important aspect of touch. If your touch has the wrong rhythm or if your instructions are unclear, you might upset her rather than uplift her. Let the rhythm of your touch be slow, firm and slightly monotonous.

FOCUS ON THE PRESENT

Help her to stay in the present and to deal with one contraction at a time. Talk about time has a negative effect. Focus on what she has done and not on what lies ahead:

– *'Now you can put that contraction on the pile of finished contractions.'*
– *'You have already dealt with those and will never have to deal with them again.'*

QUIET TIME BETWEEN RUSHES

For a woman to be brave, to go deep into her body and to follow the instructions she will need to have space to concentrate. You need to whisper and take it slowly between contractions so that she can maintain her focus. Ask 'Is it okay with you if we talk now? Let us know if we are disturbing you'. Some women like having chatter in the background, while other women cannot concentrate when surrounded by sounds. Use your communication skills and humour in these situations.

AFFIRM AND BE CLEAR

Pregnant women feel a wide array of emotions when thinking of the upcoming childbirth. Sadness, fear, anger, anxiety and happiness are just some examples. Make arrangements for how to deal with strong bursts of feeling beforehand. This will make it easier for you to take charge and help her through a particularly difficult phase. The most important thing to remember is to highlight the positive. The word 'brave' is effective and encouraging. It is not as loaded as the words 'good' or 'fantastic'. You might also want to use the word 'dare'.

– *'I know it feels difficult… but I am here and I am going to help you. Let's face the next contraction… here it is… look into my eyes… breathe… now it subsides… let it go… rest.'*
– *'You are so relaxed… keep doing what you are doing. Move your body… just like you are doing.'*
– *'You are so brave. Dare to go a little deeper, a little deeper.'*

HUMOUR

A good laugh will do wonders for the woman. Humour is a great help. Fear can make her get stuck in negative feelings. Laughing at your jokes will make her relax. She might be able to look at the situation with a little distance and humour. Childbirth is normally full of funny situations and humour is a great tool. You do not have to be a clown or a comedian, but you can highlight the funny situations and sounds. By doing so you create lightness and deepen your connection. Use the humour you and your partner already have between you.

Six principles during contractions

1. Communicate clearly
To avoid having to guess what the woman wants or if she likes what you are doing, agree in advance how you will communicate during labour. She needs to feel free without having to worry about offending or hurting someone while in labour. Simple gestures for 'yes', 'no' and 'stop' are often the most effective. One such gesture might be her lifting her hand if she has had enough.

– *'Lift your hand as soon as it doesn't feel good and I will stop.'*
– *'If you want me to stop, say stop. If I talk too much raise your hand.'*

2. Three rushes
It is very difficult to be brave and take over if you see the woman struggling. To do this you can ask her to go along with you for three

rushes. Have confidence in yourself and do not take it personally if she doesn't find your suggestions helpful. A woman I was working with had a very hard time when I first entered the room. I slowly helped her to relax and sink deeper into her body. Despite being more relaxed than before, she did not find what we were doing helpful. The pain was still there. I asked if it felt worse. It did not. I explained the difference I could see in her body as briefly and clearly as I could. After that she felt motivated to continue.

– 'I will give you a massage. If you find this disturbs you, just lift your hand. Let's try during three contractions and if it doesn't work we'll go back to doing it your way.'
– 'I will talk you through the contraction. Lift your hand if you want me to be quiet. Let's try during three contractions. After that, we can evaluate and see if it made things easier or not.'

3. The moment the rush starts

You need to catch the labouring woman right at the start of the contraction. It has to happen the moment she can sense the contraction. The reason behind this is that if you are too late, the woman might be lost in the sensation and be unable to follow your instructions. It is a good idea to use a code word like 'now', or a gesture for when the contraction starts. In this way you will be right there from the start guiding her to breathe calmly, getting heavy, using her deep voice and allowing herself to flow with her body. Remind her to signal from time to time.

- 'Simply lift you hand or say "now" when you feel the rush.'
- 'As soon as you can sense the contraction let me know by saying "now" and I'll be right there with you, guiding you.'

4. Simplify
We often try to explain ourselves using too many words or long sentences. This can be perceived as disturbing or confusing. Words are just as important as touch and should be clear and precise. Keep repeating the same words over and over again. This is more effective than using too many words.

- 'Dare to get heavy... heavy... heavy.'
- 'Relax your shoulders... relax your jaw... let your body become heavy. Relax your shoulders... relax your jaw... Let your body become heavy.'

5. Continue simplifying
Get used to sounding like a broken record player. Most labouring women need to hear an enormous amount of repetition. You might not think she wants to hear 'get heavy' any more after having heard these words for the last three hours. But if you stop she might lose her momentum or get frustrated. Imagine her stuck in a tornado. The force is great and the words are her safety harness. Keep taking her through every contraction. Be close to her and touch her.

- 'Heavy, heavy, heavy. Feel yourself getting heavier and heavier and heavier.'

– 'Relax your shoulders, let them sink down, heavy, heavy… relax your shoulders… heavy, heavy.'

6. Doing it yourself

The woman will not follow along if you only use words when instructing her. She is in a place where she will sometimes only be able to grasp physical instructions. You will also need to show her what you mean. She will not do what you tell her, but rather what you show her. Use a deep voice when you ask her to use a deep voice. If you want to encourage her to be brave and use the 'yes' word, you yourself will have to do the same.

– 'Allow yourself to make sounds. Use a deep voice. Follow me… deeeep…'

THE PARTNER'S BIRTHBAG

Bring a bag to the hospital or birthing centre. It is helpful if the birth partner is responsible for packing his or her own bag containing items for his or her own needs and also items to support the woman in labour. The contents of this bag could include:

- lavender oil
- a light blanket
- massage oil
- a torch or small battery-operated light to adjust the mood of the room

- music
- food, drinks and snacks
- hair bands
- whatever else you might think you need

AFTER THE BABY IS BORN

It is very common for the new mother to start shaking after delivery. This can also occur during labour. Shaking happens when the body seeks to restore the balance between oxygen and carbon dioxide. You can help her to reduce the shaking by cupping your hands over her mouth and nose like a mask. You can also use a towel or a paper bag. She should inhale the same air that she is exhaling. Make sure no air leaks in through any gaps. It takes about five to ten minutes to achieve full effect. It is important to keep this up for at least five minutes.

Ask for some private time after the baby is born. This is a magical moment. Do not let practicalities take over. Cover yourself and the baby with a sheet or blanket to start the bonding process if the room is messy or full of disturbing sounds.

The body releases oxytocin during a massage. This is the same hormone the mother and child release during nursing. Massaging the new mother's feet, hands and face is, therefore, a great way of helping the nursing and bonding.

Brief overview

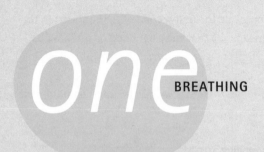

one BREATHING

Breathe *softly* and *soundlessly* throughout the entire contraction.

SUPPORT PERSON:
1. The instruction 'soundless' will help you to continuously guide the woman towards proper breathing. As soon as you can hear her breath, you move in and help her to go softer and quieter. The breathing should be soft, slow and soundless.

– *'Soooft, quiet inhale… slooowly exhale… soooft inhale… slooow, quiet exhale.'*
– *'Not so much air, soft, soundless. Breathe quietly… dare to try breathing without making a sound… that is exactly it… soooundless and soft.'*

If she struggles with the slow breathing, guide her towards a faster rhythm, but keep it soundless. I am choosing to make a point about keeping the breathing soundless and soft since it is common for it to still be audible in spite of this instruction. You might think to yourself 'well, it is pretty much soundless and she seems to be doing fine'. But try to make her breathe without sound during three rushes. It is worth it, I promise.

2. Establish how to communicate the first second of the contraction to be able to help her. This means she may raise her hand or say 'now' as soon as she feels the first ripple of a new contraction roll in.

– 'Say "now" or raise your hand as soon as you feel the contraction so that I can help you.'

End the contraction with a sigh
Finish every contraction by inhaling deeply and then sigh peacefully when exhaling. This will release any tension built up during the contraction.

SUPPORT PERSON:
1. Encourage the woman to inhale deeply, and then exhale with a sigh at the end of each contraction.

– 'The contraction is over. Fill your lungs with air and let's exhale with a soft and lovely sigh together [sigh with her].'
– 'Sigh the air out and let any tension melt away.'

2. Solidify the 'principle of repetition'. This involves you echoing every decision the two of you make. After the breathing is established, you remind her of the soundless breathing, and as each contraction wears off, you remind her of the sigh and so on. During the contraction you keep repeating your instructions over and over again.

– 'The rush is over. Help your body to relax. Fill your lungs with air and give a great sigh. Again. All you have to do is inhale and then sigh.'

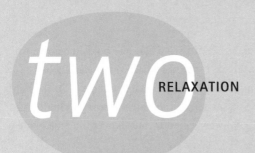

two RELAXATION

When you feel the rush coming let go of the whole body, the face, the jaw, the shoulders, the arms and the legs. Try different positions, such as standing, lying down or walking. Recall the image of sinking into water.

SUPPORT PERSON:
1. As the contraction starts, you can help the woman to get heavy. She should be like a rag doll, letting go of all extremities and all tension.

– *'The rush is coming in. Be still and lean on me. Let go and let everything sink.'*

Help the woman to let go and become heavy in her jaw, shoulders, thighs and pelvis. Use simple words while guiding her. You might find the word 'heavy' useful. Direct her with a calm, deep voice.

– *'Let go of your jaw… release your shoulders… heavy bottom and legs… let go of your jaw… release your shoulders… heavy legs…'*
– *'Heavy thighs… heavy… just be in the flow… release your jaw… let it go and let gravity take over… relax your shoulders… heavy…'*

Repeat this over and over again. Try to see where she holds tension and bring her attention to these areas. If she has a hard time relaxing her jaw, keep reminding her and direct her as to what she can do. Stroke her jaw, shoulders and brow if you see tension. If you see worry wrinkles on her forehead, lovingly and gently sweep your thumb over the area while repeating the mantra.

– *'Relax your forehead. Open up. Smooth face… heavy… release…'*

2. Establish the 'simplicity principle' by selecting a few words to repeat.

– *'Let go of your jaw, relax your shoulders, feel your weight, heavy, heavy, heavy.'*

Repeat these phrases or words over and over again using a calm, deep voice.

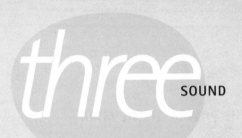

three
SOUND

Use a deep sound that resonates from your lower abdomen. The sound should be smooth and audible throughout the entire exhalation. At the end of a push close the mouth and let the sound resonate within. But do not stop sounding.

SUPPORT PERSON:

1. Help the woman find her deep, dark voice. This will engage the muscles she needs to push the baby out. Use your own voice to show her how the tone should be slow and deep.

– *'Sound as much as you want, as long as you use a deeeeep voice. Darker and deeper. Let the voice go all the way down to your belly. Deep… deeep… deeeep.'*

2. As she is in the pushing phase you can help her feel heavy and sink towards her heels or the floor. Repeat the word 'down'. 'Brave' and 'courageous' are two words that work like magic when it comes to encouraging her to access just that – her bravery and courage.

– *'Find the courage to sink towards your heels. Only think about the word down… down… down… down… you are so brave…'*

3. Establish the 'do it yourself principle'. Encourage her to use a deep, dark voice by showing her.

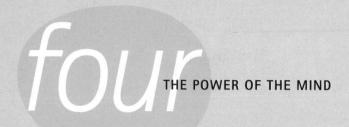

four THE POWER OF THE MIND

If you feel negative energy or thoughts take over, start saying 'yes'. Slowly say 'yes' over and over again, using your calm, deep voice.

SUPPORT PERSON:

1. If the negative energy gets too strong, or if she starts saying 'no', you can help her by saying 'yes' yourself. Use your own deep voice. Applying humour at this point is a good idea. This could be a thread through the entire birth process. Use your sense of humour and fun to make her laugh and relax.

– *'Dare to say "yes" instead of "no". During the next three contractions say "yes"… you do not have to continue if it does not feel right. Yeeeeesss… go with it… yeeeess… yeeess…'*

2. Suggest she uses 'three contractions' since more than that can feel overwhelming at first.

3. Help her by using your calm, deep voice while saying 'yes'.

Touch/massage

To reinforce the tools and lessen stress and worry, you can use massage.

Technique:
Massage or stroke starting at the shoulders and firmly bringing your hands down along her back and arms. You might also want to include foot massage in your repertoire since this is highly effective.

1. Palms open, fingers slightly apart. Massage by firmly stroking her back (most pressure on your fingers). Start at her shoulders and work down along the arms and back. Make it one long, calm and sweeping movement.

2. Cup your hands slightly. Massage by squeezing one part of her body after another, moving your hands one inch at a time. Start massaging the neck, and then move down her arms and back. You can also put your hands on her shoulders, and then pull them down in one sweeping motion towards her buttocks and hips.

3. In case you do not like any of these techniques – create your own way of massaging. Whichever technique you choose, remember to start the movement from her shoulders and work your way down her body.

Sometimes the woman does not want to be caressed or touched. My experience is that this has a lot to do with how she is touched and in what way you have body contact with her. Reflect on the advice you have been given regarding rhythm and clarity. Help her to get close to you, caress her and hold her. Try to rock, or sway with her.

- Observe where the woman holds tension and massage these areas.
- Speak with a soft, deep voice and remind her to breathe and relax.

– *'Let your shoulders go'* [massage gently].
– *'Relax your entire back'* [massage lovingly].

Butterfly massage

If the pain is in her groin you can massage this area using a tickling motion. Tickle her right by the pubic bone, above the pubic hair along the groin. You can also tickle the entire belly with sweeping motions. Ask her what feels best.

Firm pressure to the lumbar region

When the pain gets strong in the back, you can massage her sacrum. This is the bony area you can feel at the end of your back. Massage the area around the sacrum, and outline the contours with your hands. Use varied pressure.

- Press, and make small circles above the sacrum and lumbar area. Do not be afraid to use force. The pressure should be stronger than the pain.
- The pressure you apply to her back will remind her to breathe through her whole body. It will relax her shoulders, jaw and neck

and make her relaxed and heavy.

- In some cases it's the opposite – the woman is sensitive towards pressure and is uncomfortable because of it. In this case you can use the softer massage techniques.

Does it feel complicated? Do not worry. At the end of the day all you have to remember when the contractions start is this:

1. Breathe soundlessly to the rhythm of your choice when the rush emerges. As the rush subsides, exhale with a sigh one or two times.

2. Relax your face, jaw, shoulders and buttocks and let your body sink heavily towards the floor during the rush.

3. As the birth process is close to the end, and in the pushing phase, you can greet the contractions with your deep voice and a feeling of being heavy.

4. If you feel negative thoughts take over and you have a hard time being in the flow – use the mantra 'yes'. Repeat the word softly and deeply throughout the contraction.

5. Your support person can give you a sense of security and closeness by massaging you whenever and wherever you need it.

Conclusion

Fear is possibly the biggest obstacle a woman has to face when she is in labour, but, by using simple tools, she can dare to face this fear and transform the birth experience. I have emphasized the woman's inner power, and how specific tools will help the body unlock the systems it already possesses to help her to give birth.

But all this will not lead to the perfect birth, because the perfect birth does not exist. Childbirth is a process where every step is important and where every emotion is true. Just like life itself the process can be a rollercoaster ride. You will have faith, you will lose faith, and then you will regain faith. Ideals and perfection can get in the way and do not belong in the delivery room. All parts of the process are equally important. Don't have any preconceived ideas about having the perfect natural birth or having a highly medicated birth without a trace of pain. Such preconceptions are equally hampering and limiting since they are not based on humility and respect for the process and you as the human being you are.

Childbirth contains the dark, as well as the lighter aspects of a woman. Giving birth to a child carries with it an opportunity to conquer obstacles within, like low self-esteem, a mistrust in the body and indirectly towards the self.

This involves facing up to your deepest fears and all your doubts. If you understand how childbirth contains all of you, and all you carry with you, you have the opportunity to face up to these things. You can decide on the boundaries yourself. It might be opening up for a little while before asking for pain medication, but it can also be a decision to give birth completely without the aid of medicine. Every step is yours to take. You decide where you want to go, depending on how you feel at the time. There is no right or wrong way to go. It is about you trusting your ability to give birth and to grow from the experience.

Many women think they will have a mainly positive experience of pain because they have prepared before giving birth. They can then be disappointed if they have a hard time during labour, and struggle to cope with the pain. It feels unsuccessful and meaningless. I had that same feeling during my first labour, until I got the support that enabled me to move through the course of events, and access my body. I was not able to understand and make sense of what had happened until after the delivery. Then I was able to learn from the experience. As an important mental preparation, it is vital to keep in mind how the reward might be delayed.

Childbirth can be divided into two parts. The first part is when you enter into the birth and give the body access to its powers. Here you do not know why you do what you do, you simply do it. It is like running a marathon or climbing a mountain where you move forward one breath at a time, inch by inch, along with your support person. The difference is that instead of you having to force yourself to take the next step, you have to focus on giving in without fighting or pushing.

Not until you have reached the other side of the mountain, or the finishing line, will you be able to make sense of your struggles. This is when you will reap the benefits. Your inner limitations have been stretched, and your horizon has forever widened. When the birth has taken place, however it might have occurred, the consciousness at the other side will start to understand, interpret and make sense of what happened. For many women this will lead to higher self-esteem, a better capacity to embrace life for what it is and a new attitude towards the body.

The most important thing is something a woman once said to me: 'Childbirth is but a breath of all the challenges you will face afterwards. When you start your life with a growing, developing child and all the trials that brings... that is when it truly starts!'

Good Luck!

Susanna Heli

Thank you

So many women have guided me to the place where I am today, and especially the women whose births I have had the honour of witnessing. They taught me all I know, pointed me in the right direction when I was wrong, and gave me positive feedback when I did something right. I am deeply grateful for this.

A midwife who has been of great importance in helping me to find my inner powers is Cayenne Ekjordh. She led me towards this inner voice and wisdom. Her immense intuition and ability to know what I and other birthing women need to be able to have an empowering experience has greatly inspired me. I am eternally grateful! She also taught me the invaluable 'diving technique', upon which I have based many of my tools.

I also want to thank midwife Gudrun Abascal for her priceless support during my years as a doula when I explored and experimented at BB-Stockholm, a maternity ward in Sweden. Her unyielding belief in putting the woman first and letting everyone around support and secure her in every way possible has helped me to develop.

Thank you to Liisa Svensson who has helped me with the book, my ability to develop as a doula and as a human being. Gunilla Ericsson and Helena Lindgren were always by my side with their deep knowledge, humour and support. Marie Berg at the School of Midwifery in Gothenburg gave me the courage to let me teach and recognized the importance and benefits of training the midwives in supporting and strengthening women in labour. My publishers Martin Wagner and Maria Pinter at Pinter & Martin understood what I was trying to say in this book, and made me do it even better. Joanna Tisell translated the book and brought the original flow and feeling into the English version, with the help of Debbie Kennett.

Thank you Mariano Amarilla for all his help in structuring and developing this book. Without him nobody would have understood anything I was trying to say. His capacity is endless! Even though I did not always jump with joy when he shredded what I had written, I will always be infinitely thankful. He is just as much a part of this book as I am.

Viktoria Wallin, Hilda Lundgren, Eugénia Hildestrand – their unique linguistic talents have brought me closer to my own language. They showed me where I needed to fill out and take more space. They have inspired, elevated and broadened my language. My sister Heidi Karikumpu – my link to the readers. Her bravery in asking me what I wanted to say, or letting me know when she did not understand helped me to not 'muddle around' and use unintelligible words. In a clean and uncomplicated way she helped me keep track of the red thread.

Many thanks to all the women and couples who have read the book – it would not be possible without them.

Last but not least many thanks to all the midwives and nurses who have shown me priceless techniques to use during labour. I have had so much fun sharing the births with them.

With gratitude!

References

Doula UK – www.doula.org.uk
Doulas of North America – www.dona.org
Susanna Heli's website – www.confident-birth.com

Books

- Abascal, G. *Att föda* (2004). Albert Bonniers Förlag.
- Alehagen, S. *Fear, Pain and Stress Hormones During Labor* (2002). Magisteruppsats i Linköping, University Medical Dissertations No. 730, PMID 16295513.
- Antonovsky, A. *Hälsans mysterium* (1991). Natur och Kultur, Sweden.
- Balaskas, J. *New Active Birth: A Concise Guide to Natural Childbirth* (1991). Thorsons.
- Brudal, L. *Födandets psykologi* (1985). Natur och Kultur.
- England, P. & Horowits, R. *Birthing From Within* (1998). Partera Press.
- Gaskin, I.M. *Ina May's Guide To Childbirth* (2003). Bantam Dell.
- Dick-Read, G. *Childbirth Without Fear* (2012). Pinter & Martin.
- Gronlien Zetterqvist, K. *Att vara kroppssubjekt: Ett fenomenologiskt bidrag till feministisk teori och religionsfilosofi* (2002). Studia Philosophiae Religionis 23.
- Heiberg-Endresen, E. & Björnstad, N. *Fødende krefter* (1992). J.W. Cappelens Förlag.
- Kitzinger, S. *The New Pregnancy & Childbirth* (2008). Dorling Kindersley.
- Klaus, M.H., Kennell, J.H. & Klaus, P.H. *Mothering the Mother* (1996). Addison-Wesley.
- Kåver, A. *Att leva ett liv, inte vinna ett krig* (2007). Natur och Kultur.
- Lerner, M. *Psykosomatik, kroppens och själens dialog* (1999). Natur och

Kultur.
- Lundberg, U. & Wentz, G. *Stressad hjärna, stressad kropp: Om sambandet mellan psykisk stress och kroppslig ohälsa* (2005). Wahlström & Widstrand.
- Lännergren, J. m.fl. *Fysiologi* (1998). Studentlitteratur.
- Nisell, R. & Lundberg, T. *Smärta och inflammation: Fysiologi och terapi vid smärttillstånd i rörelseorganen* (1999). Studentlitteratur.
- O'Driscoll, K. & Meagher D. *Active Management of Labor* (1993). Mosby.
- Simkin, P. *The Birth Partner* (1989). The Harvard Common Press.
- Sjögren, B. *Förlossningsrädsla* (1998). Studentlitteratur.
- Uvnäs Moberg, K. *The Oxytocin Factor* (2011). Pinter & Martin.
- Waldenström, U. *Föda barn: Från naturligt till högteknologiskt* (2007). Karolinska Institutet University Press.
- Währborg, P. *Stress och den nya ohälsan* (2003). Natur och Kultur.

Articles
- Alehagen, S., Wijma, B. & Wijma, K. Fear of childbirth before, during and after childbirth. *Acta Obstet Gynecol Scand*, 2006;85:56–62.
- Alehagen, S. & Wijma, K. & Wijma, B. Fear during labor. *Acta Obstet Gynecol Scand*, 2001;80:315–320.
- Alehagen, S. m.fl. Fear, pain and stress hormones during childbirth. *J Psychosom Obstet Gynaecol*, 2005;26:3:153–165.
- Areskog, B., Uddenberg, N. & Kjessler, B. Fear of childbirth in late pregnancy. *Gynecol Obstet Invest*, 1981;12:262–266.
- Dahlberg, K. Kroppen – vår tillgång till världen. *Nord Fysio*, 1997;1:29–33.
- Eysenck, M.W. Anxiety, the cognitive perspective. *Essays in Cognitive Psychology*, 1992:35–50.
- Green, J.M., Coupland, V.A. & Kitzinger, J.V. Expectations, experiences, and psychological outcomes of childbirth: a prospective study of 825 women. *Birth*, 1990;17:15–24.

- Green, J.M. Expectations and experiences of pain in labor: findings from a large prospective study. *Birth*, 1993;20:65–72.
- Hedlund, L. & Gard, G. Tillit till den egna kroppen. *Nord Fysio*, 2000;4:67–74.
- Henry, J.P. Biological basis of the stress response. *Integr Physiol Behav Sci*, 1992;1:66–83.
- Hodnet, E.D. m.fl. Continuous support for women during childbirth. *Cochrane Database of Systematic Reviews*, 2007:3, Art. No. CDOO3766. DOI: 10.1002/14651858.CDOO3766.pub2.
- Hodnet, E.D. m.fl. Continuous support for women during childbirth. *Cochrane Database of Systematic Rewiews*, 2007:3, Art. No. CDOO3766. DOI: 10.1002/14651858.CDOO3766.pub2.
- Kennedy, H.P. m.fl. The landscape of caring for women: A narrative study of midwifery practice. *Journal of Midwifery and Women's Health*, 2004 Jan-Feb;49(1):14–23, PMID 14710136.
- Lagercrantz, H. & Slotkin, T.A. The 'stress' of being born. *Scientific American*, 1985;12:100–110.
- Lederman, R.P. m.fl. Anxiety and epinephrine in multiparous women in labor. Relationship to duration of labor and fetal heart rate pattern. *J Psychosom Obstet Gynaecol*, 1985;153:870–877.
- Lovallo, W.R. & Thomas, T.L. Stress hormones in psychophysiological research: Emotional behavioral, and cognitive implications. *Handbook of Psychophysiology*, Cambridge University Press, 1989:12–33.
- Lowe, N.K. Explaining the pain of active labor: the importance of maternal confidence. *Res Nurs Health*, 1989;12:237–245.
- McCrea, B.H. & Wright, M.E. & Myrphy-Black, T. Differences in midwifes' approach to pain relief in labor. *Midwifery*, 1998;14:174–180.
- Melender, H.L. Experiences of fears associated with pregnancy and childbirth: a study of 329 pregnant women. *Birth*, 2002;29(2):101–111.
- Melzack, R. m.fl. Labor is still painful after prepared childbirth training. *Can Med Ass J* 1981;25:357–363.

- Molin, C. & Nilsson, C.G. Stress – reaktioner och beteende. *Tandläkartidningen*, 1997;89:7.
- Saisto, T. & Halmesmäki, E. Fear of childbirth: a neglected dilemma. *Acta Obstet Gynecol Scand*, 2003;82:201–208.
- Saisto, T. m.fl. Reduced pain tolerance during and after pregnancy in women suffering from fear of labor. *Pain* 93, 2001:123–127.
- Simkin, P. Stress, pain and catecholamines in labor: Part 1. A review. *Birth*, 1986;13:227–233.
- Sjögren, B. Fear of childbirth and psychosomatic support. *Acta Obstet Gynecol Scand*, 1998;77:819–25.
- Slade, P. Expectations, experiences and satisfaction with labour. *Br J Clin psychol*. 1993;32:469-83.
- Szeverenyi, P. m.fl. Contents of childbirth-related fear among couples wishing the partner's presence at delivery. *J Psychosom Obstet Gynaecol*, 1998;19:38–43.
- Thomassen, P. m.fl. Doula – ett nytt begrepp inom förlossningsvården. *Läkartidningen* 2003;51-52:4268-4271.
- Thorstensson, S. & Nissen, E. & Ekstrom, A. An exploration and description of student midwives' experiences in offering continuous labour support to women/couples. *Midwifery*, 2007 Sep17, PMID 17881100.
- Waldenström, U. & Berman, V. & Vasell, G. The complexity of labor pain: experiences of 278 women. *J Psychosom Obstet Gynaecol*, 1996b;17:215–228.
- Waldenström, U. Experience of labor and birth in 1111 women. *J Psychosom Res*, 1999;47:471–82.
- Waldenström, U. m.fl. The childbirth experience, *Birth*, 1996;23:144–153.
- Zhang, J. m.fl. Continous labor support from labor attendant for primiparous women: A meta-analysis. *Obstet Gynaecol*, 1996;88:739–744.

also from Pinter & Martin

Childbirth Without Fear
Grantly Dick-Read

Birth Without Violence
Frédérick Leboyer

The Oxytocin Factor & The Hormone of Closeness
Kerstin Uvnäs Moberg

Birth and Sex & Rediscovering Birth
Sheila Kitzinger

Birth Matters & Ina May's Guide to Breastfeeding
Ina May Gaskin

Kiss Me! & My Child Won't Eat!
Carlos González

The Womanly Art of Breastfeeding
La Leche League International

Childbirth in the Age of Plastics & The Functions of the Orgasms
Michel Odent

The Politics of Breastfeeding & Complementary Feeding
Gabrielle Palmer

www.pinterandmartin.com